MW00448571

I am not a diabetic, but I live a low-carb lifestyle with an emphasis on diabetes prevention. I was born into a family where my father and all 13 of his siblings were Type 2 diabetics. I also have 23 firsts cousins who have diabetes. Based on my genetics, I knew I was predisposed to getting diabetes and was destined to have the same fate. I later learned that although Type 2 diabetes is a pervasive disease, it is often preventable with lifestyle modifications including exercise, weight control, and eating a healthy low carbohydrate diet. Dr. Hampton writes about removing fear providing a path to a diabetic free life simply by maintaining a low carbohydrate diet. The knowledge Dr. Hampton shares in his book provide the foundation needed to easily transition to this way of eating. By patterning my life to one where fear does not rule my thoughts and living a low-carb lifestyle, I continue to have normal diabetes tests. This should provide hope to anyone who has a family history like mine. Thank you, Dr. Hampton, for providing this valuable resource.

~Angela Willis

When I was told by Dr. Hampton that I had diabetes, I felt many emotions. I've heard many stories about how diabetes affects you. What I knew for sure was that I needed my eyes and feet to continue living the active lifestyle I was accustomed to. I was diagnosed with diabetes the summer of 2016 with a hemoglobin A1c well over 13. I was horrified and had no desire to take medication. After some consultation, I agreed to take Metformin twice daily along with a low-carb meal plan consuming less than 50 carbs daily as suggested by Dr. Hampton. I also walked my local mall 2-4 times per week. I am happy to report that within 9 months I was able to reduce my Hemoglobin A1c to 5.8 and now only take medication once daily. I really felt great after my daughter commented I had not complained about walking her college campus. That was a first. That was my affirmation that I was well on my way to overcoming diabetes. My low carb diet combined with drinking unsweetened water, tea, or coffee has given me a new lease on life. My concerns about my eyes and feet are essentially gone now that I know how to manage my diabetes.

~Linda Brothers

It finally happened! After living with diabetes for 8 years, something clicked in my brain. I knew I was not in control of my diabetes and something had to change. I think it was the combination of three things. First was the realization that both my diabetic mother and grandmother died at young ages of heart disease (just after and just before age 60 respectfully). The second was that my diabetic younger sister served as an inspiration since she was able to turn life around with lifestyle changes. Although she later died in a car accident, because of her, I knew what was possible with dietary changes. The third was finally hearing with clarity Dr. Hampton's message that if I ate properly, I could overcome diabetes. I took on the challenge of counting carbs. During my first month, I was able to loose 15 pounds. This resulted in much better control of my blood glucose values unlike I had never seen. Finally, diabetes was not in control. This was exciting since I always feared taking insulin shots. I now eat less starchy foods and avoid situations that compromise my diet.

~Delores Jones

FIX YOUR
DIET

FIX YOUR
DIABETES

FIX YOUR
DIET

FIX YOUR
DIABETES

Your Dietary Solution to Reversing Diabetes

by
TONY HAMPTON, MD, MBA,CPE

FIX YOUR DIET, FIX YOUR DIABETES

Windy City Publishers
2118 Plum Grove Road, #349
Rolling Meadows, IL 60008
www.windycitypublishers.com

Published in the United States of America

ISBN:
978-1-941478-38-7

Library of Congress Control Number:
2017934983

WINDY CITY PUBLISHERS
CHICAGO

CONTENTS

ACKNOWLEDGEMENTS

I want to personally thank many of the people who helped answer a very important question. If a book was written to help you improve your diabetes, what questions would it answer?

This question was answered by many of my patients, friends, and family who themselves struggle with diabetes. You have provided invaluable insight and your input is greatly appreciated.

This book would not have been possible without the support, inspiration, and encouragement of my wife, Karon. She is my rock and main inspiration for focusing on this condition.

As I spent time researching for my book tucked away in my home office, my children Brandon and Justin were always respectful, allowing me some time alone. Thank you for your understanding and patience through this journey. I hope I have inspired you to reach your goals. Know I will always be there to help you along your way.

I want to thank my editors for all your support. Your expertise and time provided the polishing touches I needed to make this book readable.

I want to thank the publisher for supporting my work and having the confidence to help me reach a larger audience than the patients I see.

I want to thank Judith Andre, my medical assistant at the time of this writing, whose efficiency in her role coupled with my organization's Advocate Operating System have made it possible to have the time to write this book. Together they have helped me restore the work-life balance that was previously elusive in my life. I am eternally grateful.

Finally, I want to thank my mom for creating the foundation I needed for becoming the man I am today. You modeled for me that with a little sacrifice, anything is possible.

PLEASE NOTE

I use diabetic medicines to control symptoms of diabetes.

I use a low-carb/high-fat diet to get to the root cause of Type 2 diabetes so that it can be reversed.

~Tony Hampton, MD

"What is a teacher? It isn't someone who teaches something,
but someone who inspires the student to give of her best
in order to discover what she already knows."
~Paulo Coelho

Why I Wrote This Book

I wrote this book as a work-around. So what's a work-around? It's a method for overcoming a problem or limitation in a program or system. The problem I've had is the inability to provide the education my patients need to take care of their bodies mentally, physically, and spiritually. In a healthcare system with 15-minute office visits, I've found it necessary to provide additional tools my patients need to live healthy lives. My hope is that you will read this book and use the information in it as an important resource on your journey to fixing diabetes. You have been trying to find an easy solution to preventing or controlling your diabetes and it's finally here. No complicated recipes or programs. Just a simple change in how you look at diabetes and how you will approach it moving forward.

I also wrote this book because I have realized with some reflection what my life purpose is. I enjoy teaching and have been doing just that in my clinical practice, as a parent, and periodically as a speaker. I also have a lifelong love for learning new information. I decided to take my passion for learning and teaching to help others reach their goals.

Finally, the most important aspect of my life is my family, and my wife serves as my family's anchor. When she was diagnosed with diabetes, our lives immediately changed. I made a promise to myself that I would do everything possible to help her face this disease without fear. Once fear was removed, we could work as a family to over-come this condition, never allowing it to have any significant impact on our lives. I will use continuous learning as my primary tool to take a journey with my patients, family, and readers to a new way to view-ing diabetes. A perspective where together we control our destiny as opposed to allowing diabetes to control us. I am excited for those who are willing to take this journey with me.

So if you are struggling with diabetes, you are reading the right book.

CHAPTER 1

Fix Your Motivation

"If someone is going down the wrong road,
he doesn't need motivation to speed him up.
What he needs is education to turn him around."
~Jim Rohn

Answering the WHY Question

So what is your motivation for reading this book? Is it because you feel it's time to finally win your battle with diabetes and are looking for the steps you need to take to get you there? Or is it because the world has convinced you that the reason you have this condition is because you have not taken personal responsibility for the lifestyle decisions you have made? If only you would eat less and exercise more, right? That's what you have been told for so many years and yet no matter what you do, you have not found a path to success.

I have some good news for you. You are not the problem. If that was so, we would be living in a world of unmotivated individuals un-willing to make the necessary changes to improve their overall health. I don't believe this at all. My experience with patients is that most want to be healthy and are willing to do what's needed to get healthy.

So if that's true, what's been keeping them from finding success? The answer is simple. It's not a lack of motivation but a lack of informa-tion. Yes, the path to success is understanding how our bodies work, which is becoming clearer as more and more research is being done.

In the pages of this book I will share a way of viewing your diet that perhaps no one has taught you before. With this new information you can take the steps needed to make changes in your diet and lifestyle. As you learn how to approach your food options, you will give your body access to the right nutrition. This will help you keep your blood sugars down, ultimately reducing the need for insulin, whether it comes from your pancreas (your insulin factory) or the pharmacy (medication). And yes, eating healthier can be done affordably, as long as you are open to eating some of the things you normally walk away from when shopping.

As a physician, there were times when I blamed my patients for not being at their ideal body weight until I realized one important reality. Maybe their behaviors didn't lead to their inability to process glucose biochemically, but rather their biochemistry led to the behaviors. You may want to read that last sentence again. In other words, relax and stop blaming yourself.

Once you understand how sugars affect your decisions, you will stop blaming yourself (or anyone else) for your diabetes or the effects it has on your physical condition. You will also learn that all calories are not the same and that some calories are good while others are bad.

For example, calories from sugars are not the best way to receive nutrition, no matter what you've been told about how much of your nutrition should be coming from sugars or carbs. In fact, an International Econometric Analysis of Diet and Diabetes found "sugar availability is a significant statistical determinant of diabetes prevalence rates worldwide."[1]

To put this in perspective, a 12-ounce can of regular Coke contains 39 grams of total sugar, which is about 9-1/3 teaspoons of sugar. The American Heart Association (AHA) has put together a maximum intake allowance for sugar, and according to the AHA, women should have no more than 6 teaspoons per day. Men can have up to 9 teaspoons of sugar daily. So, whether you're male or female, drinking a single 12-ounce can of Coke goes over the maximum sugar allowance for the day.[2] The average American consumes 22 teaspoons daily.

Keeping these facts in mind, it would not surprise you that drinking just one soda per day increases your risk for diabetes by 29 percent, regardless of your current weight. So I ask the question again, are you lacking motivation or lacking knowledge? I think you know the answer. Now let's start by looking at ways you can stay motivated as you work toward your goal of fixing your diabetes.

Set a Goal

The first step is to define your goal. Your short-term goal may be to get your Hemoglobin A1c under 7. Or maybe you have a long-term goal of preventing many of the complications of diabetes, like blindness or kidney failure. Either way, defining your goals will be an important step in reaching them.

Keep your goals realistic and focused. Goals that are out of reach only create an unrealistic illusion. For example, I'm a tennis fan and dream of playing at Wimbledon someday. But the reality is that I am at an age and skill level where this is an impossible dream. Likewise, if your goals are not focused, you may find yourself trying to accomplish more than your brain can handle. This results in mental fatigue, which will sap your confidence.

Now let's look at the benefits of sharing your goals.

Share Your Goal

I must admit, this is risky. Even your friends and family, who should be your greatest source of support, can sometimes be your greatest source of discouragement. Many times they are not aware that they are harming you. They want to limit your expectations so they can protect you from failure. All the same, friends and family can be our greatest ally as we work towards our goals. We want them on board when we are trying to accomplish anything, so talk to them and let them know you are determined to change and succeed. They will help keep you from falling off the wagon whenever a little motivation is needed. Your diabetes control may depend on it.

Introduce Your Goal to Your Refrigerator

In a world where stainless steel is becoming the norm, I hope I don't upset anyone with the idea of putting anything on that fancy refrigerator door. But this may be the best way to find the daily reminder you'll need to stay motivated. Most of us will pass by that big ice box at least once daily. Why not repurpose it as a reminder of your personal goals? Such a reminder could be exactly what you need to get your day started on the right foot. Consider a picture of your diabetes medicines with a big X over it. This could serve as your aspirational goal of using your diet to get off medicines.

Partner With Others to Help You Reach Your Goals

Have you ever thought, *"If only I had a life coach?"* Imagine having someone to help you as you take your journey to a place you've never been before. How secure would you feel knowing that you're not alone, but have a built-in support system to help you along the way? Partnering with someone can make this all possible.

Partnerships create an accountability that for some of us is not easily achieved alone. Not only will you benefit, but you will be returning the favor by providing the same support for the person you've created your partnership with. You are now accountable to each other, sharing both your successes and failures. Even the most successful motivational speakers, like Anthony Robbins, have life coaches. Think about the people in your circle and see if someone could fill this role in your life. If you can't find one in your circle, consider hiring a professional life coach or joining a diabetes support group in your area.

Focus on What's Important to You, Not What's Important to Others

The reality for many of us is that we spend too much time focused on other people's agendas—whether it's doing activities you really don't want to do, not knowing how to say no, or allowing others to dictate how you should live your life. The key is to reflect on your own goals and allow those goals to set your day's agenda. Once you remove distractions caused by others, there will be plenty of time to do the things that are meaningful to you.

If you rarely feel motivated, making this shift could correct your energy levels. When you're doing things for yourself, motivation will naturally be high because you're doing what your own spirit desires. Doing other people's work will never create the motivation you need to accomplish anything.

Be Careful of the Words You Use Daily

You are what you think or say you are. If you use negative words to describe yourself or your capacity to reach your goals, you will likely fulfill those negative expectations. When was the last time you recall a negative-thinking person accomplishing much or inspiring others? This doesn't happen. Understanding that our thoughts become our reality is one of the most important keys to creating an environment that fosters success. If you believe you can fix your diabetes, you will.

Create a Positive Environment to Nurture Your Spirit

I listen to inspirational messages daily. Messages from those who have mastered the art of positive thinking. They are so easy to find—in books, with an Internet search, or on Youtube. This has changed my life and it will do the same for you.

All you need to do is take a few minutes each day to get the positive juices flowing. This will enable you to counter the negative forces you will certainly face each day. Whether it's the local news, a negative co-worker, a mean boss, or an unsupportive family member, your ability to manage the negative energy they are emitting is made easier with the armor of positive thoughts in your head.

So take a moment to think about all your activities and the time and resources they use. Then start the process of removing those activities which don't add value or help you reach your goal of better controlling your diabetes. By replacing activities which don't serve you with activities that do, you will find it easier to reach your goals. Will you have the courage to take away those activities which have been part of your routine for so long? Sometimes it's what we don't do that harms us the most.

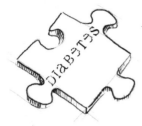

TAKEAWAYS

- **Reflect and decide WHY you are motivated to fix your diabetes. Your motivation may be a person, or it may be a goal you are trying to reach.**

- **Set a specific goal with a defined date to reach it. This could be a target level of hemoglobin A1c.**

- **Share your goal with someone who wants to help you reach it, to create accountability.**

- **Write your goal on a sticky note and place it on your refrigerator as a daily reminder.**

- **Get yourself a life coach.**

- **Focus on your own priorities and not the priorities of others.**

- **Speak encouraging language to yourself and others.**

- **Make sure your day is started with positives messages.**

CHAPTER 2

FIX YOUR BELIEF SYSTEMS

"Your beliefs become your thoughts,
Your thoughts become your words,
Your words become your actions,
Your actions become your habits,
Your habits become your values,
Your values become your destiny."
~Mahatma Gandhi

What Are Our Beliefs?

A belief is the state of mind in which a person thinks something is the case, without there being empirical evidence to prove that this particular thing is the case with factual certainty. In other words, belief is when someone thinks something is reality, or true, even when the person has no absolute verified foundation for the certainty of the truth or realness of that thing.[3]

Why Do I Believe the Things I Believe?

I am amazed at how much influence we as parents have over our children. We have the capacity to indoctrinate them into believing almost anything we desire. Not until my children asked about all the Amazon boxes their gifts came in did we finally tell them the truth about Santa Claus. My children never questioned their belief in Santa Claus because they had no reason to doubt us, their parents, who they trusted completely.

In fact, most of our beliefs are never challenged. Why would we want to question the things we have learned from our parents, teachers, friends, and family? If we can't trust them, then who can we trust? However, it's important that we have a questioning attitude and do not just accept things at face value. I suggest the adage, "trust but verify."

This will remove the need to believe things just because they make us feel secure or good. Allowing different perspectives to emerge will help fix old beliefs that simply don't work in our lives anymore. The sooner you let go of false beliefs, the sooner they will stop having power over you.

Fix What's Holding You Back

Just when you thought you had it all figured out, life shows you that maybe you need to think about things a little differently. Maybe that's the reason you picked up this book in the first place. You are searching for the answer to a simple question: How do I fix my diabetes?

Maybe you know someone who seems to be doing a better job living with this challenging condition. Or maybe you believe there's a cure. When you hear such stories, even though it gives you hope, you have struggled to take the next step of making this your reality. So what's holding you back? What's keeping you from accomplishing what could be so important in your life?

- Is it your lack of self-confidence?

- Lack of knowledge of the steps needed to be successful?

- Are you simply too busy to make YOU your number one priority?

I suggest all these and more can be factors. But the one thing I know holding many people back is how they think, why they think what they think, and not being able to change when thinking differently is needed.

If you are only a reflection of your life experiences, then how can you use those experiences to help you reach your short—and long-term goals? You can't change what has happened in the past. You do, however, have complete control over what happens next. You have started that journey by reading this book. People who are successful are always searching for the truth. They never settle for following the herd. Their intuition tells them that there is something out there, they just need to find a way to uncover the answer. Reading this book will do the same for you in your fight against diabetes.

You say you need a life coach? I have an idea. Consider me your diabetes life coach. I'll help you finally take control of this condition. Together we'll remove many of the fears you have about diabetes.

But remember, this partnership is not the key. The key is your ability to change how you view your life experiences. This will empower you to change your entire attitude, because for the first time you have hope that something inside of you will be all you'll need to get to your goals. You now control your destiny, not because you have learned how to use your experiences, but because YOU are no longer a victim of your circumstances.

You have all the power. Use it.

Take Away the Power from the Past

How do we prevent our life experiences from harming us? I would like to say it's easy, but in reality changing how you view the world is not a simple task. The good news is that it becomes a lot easier when you are able to separate experiences that harm you from those that don't.

We don't need to completely eliminate the bad experiences, because they provide an opportunity for us to grow or see things in another way. So taking a moment to repeat experiences that help you and learning from those that don't is the key. The truth is successful people have just as much negative baggage as those who are less successful. But they've learned to view negative experiences as lessons learned and never use them as excuses.

When I pledged Alpha Phi Alpha fraternity in college I was asked to recite the following quote, "Excuses are tools of incompetence used to build monuments of nothing. For those who specialize in them shall never be good at anything else."

These words may be hard to read, but must be lived by. The young men who pledged us seemed harsh, but they knew we had something inside of us that would help us overcome any obstacle. In those days we were attempting to balance school, personal life, and fraternity priorities, which at times seemed impossible. Fearing that my grades would suffer, I questioned whether pledging was the right thing to do, especially since I realized my grades would be so vital for me to get into medical school. But there was something inside me that allowed me to prevail and overcome all the obstacles I faced during those difficult years of college. There was something inside providing the inspiration I needed to carry on.

That same something is inside all of us. Yes, it's inside you as well. You just need to channel it when times get tough. Sometimes a simple reminder is enough. At other times it requires some deep reflection. Either way, it's there. And once you realize it, you can use it to reach your goals. Now let's move on to a simple question you need to ask yourself.

Are Your Current Beliefs Still Serving You?

We are all a reflection of our life journey. That journey has shaped how we perceive the world we live in. Knowing your thoughts have been shaped this way should cause you to pause and wonder:

- Is the foundation that makes me who I am a strong one?

- Was it built on factual information or on untruths and superstitions?

Although it may be impossible to completely distinguish between the two, there may be another way to approach this problem. How about simply analyzing whether or not a belief you have is helping you achieve all you desire in life. By asking this simple question, you may discover that many of the things you take for granted need to be reconsidered.

For example, I once felt that my children needed a hearty meal right after school. The reality, however, was that this led to tired children with no energy left to complete their homework after eating. After consulting with a friend who happened to work in education, my wife and I tried a little experiment. We gave our children a light healthy snack after school instead of that hearty meal. We simply saved the healthy meal for a little later.

The result was amazing. Although they complained at first, having the courage to change our old belief system resulted in two energetic boys now able to alertly complete their homework. We immediately saw an improvement in their performance, as well as less stress in our home. Gone were the days where we spent half the evening trying to keep them awake. We learned from this experience that we should never be afraid to question old beliefs. A world of possibilities opens up when we are willing to do so.

Why FEAR is the Number One Reason Beliefs are Never Challenged

The Oxford English Dictionary defines fear as an unpleasant emotion caused by the belief that someone or something is dangerous, likely to cause pain, or a threat. My favorite acronym to define fear is: FEAR is False Evidence Appearing Real.

I could give many examples of why we do things that are not supported by reasonable evidence. For example, I still have conversations with patients about their FEAR of using insulin. Many of my patients connect the use of insulin to the many complications related to diabetes. It is *delaying* the use of insulin, however, that leads to the very complications they fear. Ironically, they avoid using the medicine that could help prevent what they fear.

So what's the number-one cause of preventable death in the United States? It's tobacco use. But I would argue that FEAR should rank just as high, since so many people with real medical problems never get the help they need due to unfounded fears. Don't let that be you. Remove FEAR from your life.

Focus on Reducing the Number of Limiting Beliefs You Have

Limiting beliefs refer to the thoughts and/or stories you tell yourself that prevent you from living in your authentic power. Limiting beliefs impact the choices you make and how you behave in any given situation.

Why would anyone want to hold on to something that limits their ability to be the very best they can be? The struggles we face in life are difficult enough without letting negative beliefs restrict our progress. Start reflecting on how you view yourself. How do you talk to yourself? When things get tough, do you tell yourself you can overcome any obstacle in front of you, or do you say the opposite? Either way, you're right.

Finding the positive voice within you gives you all the power. You must counter all the negative messages you receive throughout the day with positive ones. I start my day listening to various motivational speakers sharing messages of encouragement. This gives me the ammunition to counter any negative thoughts, people, or circumstances I may face.

Keep in mind that this will not only help you face your day but may have a significant impact on the people who come in contact with you. Yes, you have the power to brighten their day with your positive energy. What a gift to give your family, co-workers, or even the strangers you meet on the street.

Simply replace limiting beliefs with limitless beliefs. This will empower you and free you from the shackles of negativity, which have kept you from reaching your goals. How different would our world be if everyone began their day with positive affirmations? It will take one person at a time, starting with you. Why not now? Why not you? It's time for you to be the author of your own story. With pen and pad in hand, start writing the story you can be proud of. You have a best-selling novel in your hand, and you will be the main character. I can't wait to see how your story goes.

Fixing Old Beliefs Requires Getting Out of Your Comfort Zone

Many people don't want to change because they have always done things a certain way and aren't ready to step off a familiar path. But if success is what you are looking for, you must be open to change. Your circumstances won't change until you change. It's just that simple.

Imagine this scenario. Are you known in your family as the one who can really cook up a tasty holiday meal? What if you have always added salted to your vegetables when you cooked them, but later learned that cooking with too much salt greatly increased your risk of heart disease? Are you willing to risk your cooking reputation and use alternatives so you can live the healthier lifestyle you want?

This would be a leap for many people, but if you don't take that leap you will never know what's possible. It's not about living up to other people's expectations—it's about making *you* your number one priority. Do you love yourself enough to do that? I love you even though I have never met you, and I know the power you have within you.

Now that you understand that your life experiences affect your beliefs, the question becomes, what do you need to do to make sure those experiences don't become a barrier to how you deal with diabetes? I think it's time to look at your routines.

Routines

It's now time to look at your routines to determine how they have affected you. Your routines are the foundation for your whole day.

They are the building blocks for what's to come later. Are your routines building a strong foundation for you to accomplish what you want to do? Or are they barriers, making your goal less likely to be achieved?

As I have moved towards a more healthy lifestyle, I have found there were many things I was doing that literally sabotaged my ability to be productive. For example, being a sports fan, I was devoted to watching my favorite sports team, the Chicago Bulls. When they played teams on the West coast, their games started later in the evening. Even knowing that I needed to wake up as early as 5:30 a.m., I would still stay up late to watch the end of the game. How INSANE is that? My new routine is to watch Youtube full game highlights of the Chicago Bulls. This satisfies my appetite to see all the plays of the game which can be done in less than 10 minutes. The time I have saved with this approach is amazing.

So ask yourself, are your routines helping you or hurting you? How do you start your day? Is it by pressing the snooze button multiple times because you didn't go to bed on time? Are you always stressed in the morning, running late because you didn't do the proper preparation? Are you exercising in the morning to get the juices flowing? When you get in the car to drive to work are you listening to music with negative lyrics or some DJ sharing celebrity gossip which adds little to your life or spirit? Instead, why not listen to a motivational speaker whose words fill you with the encouragement to get through your busy day. Your routine matters. It's time to reflect on it and find one that helps you reach your full potential.

Making the Needed Changes

You have now reflected on your life experiences and routines. So what's the next step? If those experiences and routines are not helping you get the most out of life, it's time to make changes. It's not as hard as you think, since change needs to be done step by step.

In life, change does not have to be done in an instant. It's okay to exercise a little patience and let it happen slowly over time. Reading this book may provide some tips you want to act on and change suddenly, but the hard work of changing your behaviors requires more patience. In fact, research suggests that on average it takes 66 days to acquire a new habit. So give yourself at least that much time before you expect any changes you are thinking about making to become your new reality.

Organizing Your Plan

When you're ready to make change happen, you need to organize your priorities. Ask yourself these questions:

- What do you want to accomplish?

- Is your goal to get off insulin?

- Do you want to take fewer medicines?

- Are you having diabetic complications you hope to reverse?

- Do you want to cut back on the number of times you need to check your blood sugars?

Whatever your situation, write down what you are trying to accomplish so that you know where you are going.

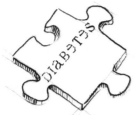

TAKEAWAYS

- Make a pledge that nothing from the past will hold you back from reaching your goals.

- Recognize that we all have the internal motivation to be successful—we just have to learn how to channel it.

- Analyze whether or not a belief you have is helping you achieve all you desire in life.

- Don't allow FEAR to paralyze you and keep you from taking action.

- Reflect on your beliefs and replace limiting beliefs with limitless beliefs.

- Be willing to get out of your comfort zone.

- Evaluate your routines to make sure they are building a strong foundation for you to accomplish what you want to do.

- Give yourself at least two months to allow any changes you are making to become routine.

- Write down your plan to keep you organized and focused.

CHAPTER 3

FIX YOUR KNOWLEDGE ABOUT DIABETES

"All truths are easy to understand once they are discovered;
the point is to discover them."
~Galileo Galilei
The father of modern science

Type 1 and Type 2 Diabetes and Beta Cells

Diabetes has been known since around the first century B.C.E., when a Greek physician, Aretaeus the Cappadocian, named it *diabainein*, meaning "a siphon," or "to pass through," referring to the excessive urination associated with the disease. The actual word diabetes was first recorded in 1425, and in 1675, the Greek word *mellitus*, meaning "like honey," was added to the name, to reflect the sweet smell and taste of the patient's urine. Now I've been known as a dedicated physician since my early training days: I have worked at county hospitals with limited resources, delivered over 10 babies in one night, and spent many nights as a resident on call with no sleep. But never have I been asked to taste the urine of my patients to determine if they were diabetic. I have nothing but respect for the many clinicians who once used this method to diagnose this condition.

While all this provides some interesting trivia, what's really important is understanding how this disease works so we can defeat it. Let's begin by differentiating between the two types of diabetes.

Type 1 diabetes was once called insulin-dependent diabetes, while Type 2 was non–insulin-dependent. This terminology was changed however, since so many Type 2 diabetics eventually become insulin-dependent. To understand either type, you must understand how the pancreas works.

The pancreas is a gland just under our left ribs which is responsible for producing insulin. Within it can be found the islets of Langerhans, which contains beta cells. Beta cells produce insulin in response to the glucose we ingest. This insulin then travels into the bloodstream en route to various cells in the body.

All cells need glucose as a source of energy, which is why they have insulin receptors. When insulin binds to the cell receptors, it serves as a key to allow glucose into the cell, providing the energy needed for the cell to carry out its specific function. When this process works well, the body functions as it should. The reality for too many people is that the process does not go well. Thus the need for books like this to find a way to fix what is not working.

Type 1 Diabetes

Type 1 diabetes occurs when things don't go as planned. With Type 1 diabetes, the beta cells are somehow destroyed within the islets of Langerhans of the pancreas. Beta cell destruction results in no insulin production, and as a result no way to get glucose into the various cells that need it. You may then ask a very important question. Why would a normally functioning beta cell suddenly lose its ability to function properly? A few theories have been posed.

Theory #1: An autoimmune process has occurred. Autoimmune implies self-destruction. In other words, your body mistakes the beta cells for foreign cells and attacks them. The next logical question is, why would the body destroy itself? It probably wouldn't unless it felt threatened or did not realize it was destroying itself. This is exactly what is speculated to be happening. It is thought that various viruses, including possibly mumps or measles, have proteins on their surfaces that look like the proteins on the beta cells in the pancreas. The immune system does not like foreign viruses, so it creates antibodies to destroy the viruses. In this case, if the beta cells look like the viruses your immune system is attacking, they become an accidental victim. This can occur suddenly and without warning.

Unfortunately, many of the proposed viruses that look like beta cells occur in children, which may be one of the reasons we see Type 1 diabetes in children.

Theory #2: Early exposure to cow's milk protein may cause a similar reaction, since these proteins look very much like those found in beta cells. Since this is the primary source of nutrition in many countries, there should be no surprise that this theory would lead us to expect a high number of cases of diabetes in countries where milk consumption is high.

If either of these theories is true, we may have some opportunities to decrease the number of people who acquire Type 1 diabetes. This could be done by improving the immunization success rate, which would decrease the number of people who get illnesses that are likely to result in this type of immune response.

Type 2 Diabetes

Type 2 diabetes is a disease of *insulin resistance*. The islets of Langerhans and their beta cells are okay. But the body's other cells are not receiving the proper message, so glucose is prevented from entering them. Some have theorized this is due to inflammation causing disruption in the messaging process. As a result, glucose can't get into the cells, resulting in high glucose levels in the bloodstream. Beta cells respond by producing more insulin. More and more insulin is produced, until the message to allow glucose into the cell is strong enough to overcome what is essentially a dysfunctional messaging system. Over time, high glucose levels results in higher insulin production.

With so much demand for insulin, the beta cells eventually burn out, losing their ability to keep up the needed insulin production. Unless the cycle is reversed, Type 2 diabetes will continue to progress until all the beta cells have burned out, eventually resulting in no insulin production. This is when Type 2 diabetics become dependent on external sources of insulin. This is the outcome of insulin resistance.

Fix Your Insulin Resistance

INSULIN'S JOB

Insulin has a very important role in our bodies. It gets much-needed energy into our cells as glucose. Without this energy source, our ability to provide our bodies with the energy to function would be short-lived. But insulin's job does not end there.

Do you know what happens when you drink a soda? Soda usually contains on average 9.5 teaspoons of sugar, and chances are you don't need all that sugar as an energy source. But don't worry, that extra sugar won't go to waste, because insulin has the job of storing the energy as glycogen in your muscles and liver, and as fat in the rest of the body. How lucky we are to have insulin for this important function?

The problem for many of us is that the need for this stored form of glucose is limited, since so many of us don't actually become active enough to use it at some future date. As a result, many of us have a cycle of continued fat storage, which ultimately results in obesity. Even worse, as we accumulate more of this fatty tissue in our body, we become more and more resistant to insulin. It's as if your body is screaming, we have enough fat storage so we are closing down the storage bins. At that point it doesn't allow our bodies to store any more glucose.

The problem is that your pancreas did not get that memo. It continues to crank out more and more insulin, attempting to overcome this resistance. What results is a hyper-insulin state. This would be okay if insulin was a harmless hormone, but the reality is that when it is overproduced, insulin can be harmful, and it usually is. Insulin is a growth hormone, and too much growth hormone will make things grow.

In the case of our bodies this can lead to increased risk of colon cancer; eating foods with a high glycemic index increases that risk by 70 percent. Further research shows that eating this way will also triple the risk of coronary artery disease. So the goal would be to avoid foods that have a high glycemic index, since eating them will lead to insulin spikes. This is not as hard as you may think, since we know which foods predict an increased risk of diabetes.

INSULIN RESISTANCE AND HOW TO REVERSE IT

Now that you understand that Type 2 diabetes is about insulin resistance, it's time to rethink how you are approaching your treatment for this condition. Most doctors and their patients focus on reducing the blood glucose values and if they're successful they feel they're controlling diabetes. But I asked myself if we were fixing the core problem or simply treating the symptoms. After reflecting on the question, I realized the core problem may not be elevated blood glucose levels after all. High glucose values are simply a symptom of diabetes. So where should the focus be?

The answer is insulin resistance. By focusing on this, you could achieve much better results, since this is essential to fixing your diabetes. Let's use an analogy to help think about this concept in a different way. If I see a patient who presents with a painful throat, red and swollen tonsils, swollen lymph nodes in the neck, and a fever, I know I likely have a patient who needs to be treated for strep throat. In order to solve his problem, I will need to give him an antibiotic to fight the bacteria that is causing his symptoms. If I gave this patient Tylenol, I would only be treating his symptoms, and would likely end up with a patient who feels better but isn't really cured.

This is what we are doing with our diabetes treatment. This is also likely the reason we consider this a progressively worsening disease. By shifting your focus, you will find a path to the solution you've been searching for. Why focus on insulin resistance? Because when insulin levels are high due to resistance, lipolysis (fat breakdown) is inhibited, sensitive arteries throughout the body are exposed to damaging higher levels of glucose, muscle protein synthesis is reduced, and glycogen-filled cells are converted to fat for storage.

So How Do We Get Insulin to Start Working Better Instead of Simply Continuing the Old Approach of Increasing Insulin Levels?

The first step is to realize that as we take more and more insulin, the body will become more and more resistant, as is the case with any other drug you use in excess. Your body simply becomes more tolerant to the insulin your pancreas is producing, making the need for more insulin production even greater. When you then consider that insulin may actually increase your weight gain (since it is the fat storage hormone), which in turn increases your need for insulin, you will find yourself in a vicious cycle that must be broken in order to find the diabetes control you are seeking.

So the fundamental message of this book is that insulin resistance is more a dietary disease than anything. That's why a dietary fix is more logical than using more and more medication. Excessive insulin has negative effects that include obesity, high triglycerides, low HDL, hypertension, heart disease, cancer, periodontitis, and fatty liver.

Even so, I caution anyone reading these words that medications—including insulin—provide a life-preserving bridge from where you are currently to where you want to be. Keep in mind that insulin has very important functions in our bodies and is not the enemy at normal levels. We need insulin to live and without it we would not last very long. So as you journey to a life where your body's insulin resistance is lowered, continue to use medication in partnership with dietary changes until you have reached your goal of a reduced need for medication.

Now let's learn some of the approaches to reversing insulin resistance.

Ways to Lower Your Insulin Resistance

BARIATRIC SURGERY

Diabetes is one of the top ten causes of death in the United States. And its most controllable risk factor is obesity. Reducing the incidence of this disease could be done by simply tackling obesity, since approximately 90 percent of Type 2 diabetes mellitus (T2DM), the most common form of diabetes, is attributable to excessive body fat.

Now consider this. The American Society of Metabolic and Bariatric Surgery states that, "metabolic and bariatric surgery is the most effective treatment for Type 2 diabetes among individuals who are affected by obesity and may result in remission or improvement in nearly all cases." Of all the treatments for Type 2 diabetes, including my favorite (lifestyle interventions), bariatric surgery is the clear winner.

Nearly 90 percent of patients who have bariatric surgery see improved blood glucose values as well as reductions in medications and diabetes-related health problems. There is also a 78 percent diabetes remission rate, with a return to normal blood glucose values. This eliminates the need for diabetes medications in many cases. With such a high success rate, this modality should be considered for any patient who is overweight and has not been successful with other interventions.

INTERMITTENT FASTING

There is a way to mimic the benefits of bariatric surgery: fasting. When bariatric surgery is done, it is essentially a forced fast. It's clear that restricting the amount of calories that are consumed will have the expected outcome of weight loss. Intermittent fasting is a non-invasive way to achieve the same goals as surgery without the risks of having surgery. Doing this will increase insulin sensitivity, resulting in overall improvement in glucose control. When the pancreas is given a break, it has the opportunity to recover, resulting in less insulin resistance. Intermittent fasting also allows time for the stored glycogen in the liver and muscles and fat to be broken down and burned off.

LOW GLYCEMIC INDEX DIET WITH FEWER REFINED CARBOHYDRATES

Carbohydrates (carbs) become glucose when broken down by digestion. Glucose in our diets results in higher insulin levels. With excess
carbohydrates, insulin resistance can worsen. So when you minimize
carbs in your diet, controlling your diabetes becomes much easier. In
fact, suggesting that a diabetic eat a high-carb diet is like suggesting
an alcoholic have a little alcohol with each meal. It simply does not
make sense when there are lower-carb alternatives to choose from.
Keep in mind that there are many other factors which should help
you as you decide which carbohydrates are best for you. Consider the
following as you decide which carbohydrates to ingest.

CARBOHYDRATE ABSORPTION RATES

As you may know, the carbs of today are not the carbs of the past.
The refining and processing procedures during food manufacturing
have a big impact on the absorption rate of a food. As an example,
the less refined steel-cut oatmeal will take longer to absorb than the
instant oatmeal most of us are more accustomed to eating. As was
the case when you switched from white bread to 100 percent whole
wheat, it won't take long for you to become accustomed to the slight
difference in texture. The hard part may be making sure your grocery
store has what you are shopping for. Many of my patients live in food
deserts. This is an urban area where it is difficult to buy affordable or
good-quality fresh food.

CARBOHYDRATE FIBER CONTENT

Not all carbs have the same amount of fiber. For example, a sweet
potato has more fiber than a white potato. When given an option,
always try to eat the higher fiber option.

CARBOHYDRATE FORM

Yes, how your carbohydrate is shaped can make all the difference in
the world. Imagine simply purchasing a long-grain rice instead of a

short-grain rice. That simple decision could help reduce the impact rice will have on your blood glucose levels.

CARBOHYDRATE RIPENESS

Green bananas anyone? Most of us are aware that the riper the banana, the sweeter the taste. Well it does not just affect your taste buds but your blood glucose values as well. So when possible, avoid overall ripe bananas when making your smoothies or having a morning breakfast and use less ripe fruit when possible. The ripeness of food can also affect the absorption rate.

Other Lifestyle Factors

HIGHER FAT DIET

Fats slow down the digestion process and may reduce the speed at which carbs are digested. The other advantage, and possibly the most important, is that high-fat foods don't significantly raise the blood glucose levels. This not only reduces the need for insulin but also reduces the worsening of insulin resistance.

HIGHER FIBER DIET

Fiber protects against rising insulin by slowing the digestion of carbs. Fiber does this by slowing down the emptying of your stomach and the absorption of sugars and starches. Fiber is definitely an easy way to reduce the impact of carbs. This is another reason to avoid refined/processed grains, because they have been stripped of much of their fiber.

AVOID PROCESSED FOODS

Processing removes the fiber and fat from foods, which reduces the nutritional value as well as the benefits described in the previous sections. In particular, processed food tends to be absorbed quickly, resulting in faster elevation of blood glucose levels.

A comparison between table sugar and flour/cornmeal is all that's needed. Two tablespoons of flour or cornmeal is equivalent in carbs to 1 tablespoon of sugar. That's because highly refined grains like flour, when they go through the milling process, lose the parts of the wheat that slow down the digestion process. You are left with the starch, which is the part that raises your blood glucose. I usually recommend that diabetics use lower carbohydrate alternatives like coconut flour to replace white/wheat flour, and flax seed meal to replace cornmeal.

AVOID FRUCTOSE

Fructose is the sugar found in many fruits. When eaten in its natural form, it does no harm, since natural fruit contains both fiber and a more modest amount of fructose. In its more refined state, however, many researchers feel it may be one of the most damaging aspects of our diets. Stick to eating whole foods the way they were created. Fruit, for example, has plenty of water and fiber, and low density of energy. It is also impossible to overeat. Therefore eating fructose in excess isn't possible when it's still in the fruit.

Extracting fructose is a totally different situation and does cause many negative effects. These effects include:

- Worsening insulin resistance.

- Deposition of fat in the liver, where fructose is processed.

- Increased calorie ingestion, since fructose doesn't affect satiety (fullness).

- Causes the hormone that controls appetite (leptin) to be resistant.

- Has addictive properties.

The good news again is that as long as fructose is eaten in its natural form as fruit, it's totally okay. Only when it's extracted and concentrated does it become a problem.

DRINK WATER

The best thing about water is that it increases satiety (fullness) while also helping to boost your metabolic rate. If you want to control your weight as well as your diabetes, try drinking water half an hour before meals. This will result in a feeling of fullness so that when you eat you will eat less.

SLEEP

Yes, getting your "beauty" rest is important. Why? Because when you are sleeping, so is your pancreas. Sleep actually lowers insulin levels. A study done at the University of Chicago revealed some of the benefits of sleep for a diabetic. This study of young healthy men revealed that when the study subjects only got four hours of sleep for six nights, they developed early signs of diabetes in just one week. This was thought to be related to increased cortisol levels due to the stress of not sleeping. The study participants also reduced their ability to absorb glucose into their bodies' cells by 40 percent, resulting in elevated blood glucose levels. When the same men were allowed to sleep eight to ten hours for six days, all the glucose abnormalities returned to the normal levels.

Another study showed that reduced sleep resulted in insulin resistance. So remember that getting enough sleep will be just as important as the other tips offered in this book.

VINEGAR

How many times has my mom suggested something as simple as adding vinegar or vinegar-rich salad dressing to help improve my health? It turns out she was right. Vinegar increases insulin sensitivity, especially when added to a carbohydrate-rich meal.

GREEN TEA
Increases insulin sensitivity.

LIFTING WEIGHTS
Increases insulin sensitivity.

DAILY WALKING
Increases insulin sensitivity.

MEDITATION AND STRESS REDUCTION
Stress can raise cortisol levels, resulting in elevation of blood glucose levels.

LOVE FOR SOMEONE SPECIAL
Increases oxytocin levels. A study by Chinese and American scientists found that oxytocin reversed insulin resistance and improved glucose tolerance in obese mice. Another benefit of this "love hormone" is that if your body gets a surge of oxytocin when you touch or see someone, you will love that person. Oxytocin is also important in promoting trust, as well as in calming fears and reducing anxiety.

SUPPLEMENTS
Here's a list of supplements I have found helpful over the years to better control your diabetes. Keep in mind, there is no need to overdo it. Decide which supplements you want to incorporate into your lifestyle. And never forget that diet, exercise, rest, and stress reduction are even more important.

- Chromium 200-1000mg: Increases insulin sensitivity.

- Magnesium: potentiates insulin to work at the cellular level. Found in foods like leafy greens, spinach, nuts, seeds, dark chocolate, or halibut.

- Vitamin D: Deficiency associated with insulin resistance.

- Green Tea extract: Improves insulin sensitivity.

- Cinnamon: Cinnamon supplements lowered blood glucose levels in people with Type 2 diabetes in a small well-controlled study by Ting Lu and colleagues. Nutrition Research, published online June 14, 2012.[7]

- Alpha Lipoic acid: Improves insulin sensitivity and decreases insulin resistance.

- Cook with Ginger: Ginger can lower blood sugar in people with Type 2 diabetes, according to a new study by researchers from Shahid Sadoughi University of Medical Sciences in Yazd, Iran.

- Cook with Garlic: A study published in the Journal of Medicinal Food found that garlic was highly effective in increasing your insulin content in the body as well as improving glucose tolerance.

- Turmeric with black pepper: Black pepper improves bioavailability. A study from Chinese researchers found that daily supplementation with compounds found in the spice turmeric can improve blood sugar levels in people who have Type 2 diabetes. Curcumin, a major component of turmeric, is the ingredient that people most associated with providing health benefits.

- Vitamin K2 improves insulin sensitivity.

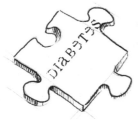

TAKEAWAYS

- Focus on eating high-fiber, low-glycemic-index foods.

- Eat more mono—and poly-unsaturated fats.

- Eat more fish high in omega 3 and more lean meats.

- Eliminate as much as possible refined/processed carbs, sugars, and sodas from your diet.

- Drink plenty of water.[8] Review the healthy beverage guideline published by Harvard and you will see that water is the clear winner. It also does a great job of curbing your appetite, with no calories to worry about.

CHAPTER 4

FIX YOUR KNOWLEDGE OF INTERMITTENT FASTING

"Fasting is the greatest remedy—the physician within."
**~Paracelsus,
One of the three fathers of Western medicine**

In order to fix your diabetes, insulin sensitivity must be improved, which is exactly what happens when you fast. With fasting, insulin sensitivity improves and the levels of insulin your pancreas needs to produce drop significantly. This is very important, not only to help control your blood glucose levels, but also to help burn fat in your body as a source of energy. Fasting can lower your blood glucose values by 3 to 6 percent, and lower your fasting insulin levels by 20 to 31 percent.[13]

Intermittent Fasting Defined

Let's start by defining what intermittent fasting is. Simply put, it's an eating pattern that cycles between periods of fasting and eating. Another way of looking at it is simply changing when you eat. You don't need to change your diet at all in order to receive its benefits.

Now of course I expect and hope you will also make dietary changes as well, since a reduction in your insulin resistance due to dietary changes will also net you great benefits. Combining this with intermittent fasting, however, may be the best way to achieve your goals.

So why are many people discovering intermittent fasting? It's because they have discovered that they can lose weight as well as improving their overall health. This has been proven with many studies, including one published by the US National Library of Medicine National Institutes of Health entitled *Fasting: Molecular Mechanisms and Clinical Applications*. Its conclusion states, "there is great potential for lifestyles that incorporate periodic fasting during adult life to promote optimal health and reduce the risk of many chronic diseases, particularly for those who are overweight and sedentary."[9]

We also must remember that most diets don't really work, primarily because as you diet your body will slow down its metabolism. As you cut calories, your metabolism will also slow down. Simply put, your body wants to maintain its current weight and will slow your metabolism down if you attempt to lose weight.

So with that in mind, let's look at some of the ways fasting can be incorporated into your lifestyle. Your goal is to find the way that best suits who you are and your needs. Keep in mind that these are time-tested approaches which many people have used with success. We are now aware that this approach is very beneficial to diabetics. You are not reinventing the wheel when trying these fasting approaches.

THE 16/8 METHOD (A.K.A. LEANGAINS)

When I wrote this book, my goal was to live every recommendation I was making. I did this so that I could personally speak to and support what I was recommending. By far, this approach to fasting was the easiest for me to follow.

The 16/8 fasting method simply involves skipping breakfast and only eating during an eight-hour window. Whether you decide to eat between 2 p.m. and 10 p.m., or 12 p.m. and 8 p.m., as long as there is a 16-hour fast, that's all that is needed. This is a lifestyle change for most who take this approach and is done most days of the week. It you choose, it's okay to take a break over the weekend.

Many of my patients were doing some variation of fasting already, but simply did not fast for a long enough period of time. For example, they would skip lunch. But skipping lunch doesn't provide enough time between meals to allow for fat breakdown. What's particularly nice about skipping breakfast instead is that many of us have very predictable lives, working 9 to 5 jobs with time set aside for lunch breaks. Keeping the same fasting approach each day makes it easier to remember and and also allows your body to become accustomed to when you will be eating. This reduces the roller-coaster appetite variations that can occur when your diet is unpredictable.

Of course, schedules do and will change, making sticking to a specific routine more challenging. But the discipline learned from routine can be just as valuable. The goal is to choose an eating time window that is both good for you socially and timed so that you are able to have a meal after exercise. Experiment with different approaches like eating dinner and breakfast if you like to exercise in the am. Either way, this approach could quickly get you on the path to not only controlling your diabetes but helping you to lose weight as well.

24-HOUR FAST (A.K.A. STOP EAT STOP)

I have always been surprised by how many of my patients don't eat breakfast and find that eating once per day is a lot easier than they expected it to be. This approach may seem difficult, but keep in mind that, unlike the 16/8 method, this approach only requires eating this way one to three times per week.

The goal is to keep dinner-time consistent so your body has a true 24-hour fast, which is what you are aiming for. I find this is easier to do on my busier days, when I am too busy to eat anyway. I also like doing this type of fast during the week. Being at work reduces the temptations found at home and the risk of making bad choices. Not only will your pancreas thank you for giving it a break for 24 hours, but so will your waistline. Remember that insulin is the fat storage hormone and by greatly reducing the need for insulin during fasting there is no need for insulin production and as a result no fat storage.

Unlike the 16/8 method, the 24-hour fast is more adaptable to many lifestyles. If I know I am having a business lunch, I simply don't fast that day. Whether the fasts are done back-to-back or are spread out throughout the week is totally determined by convenience. There are no rules to follow other than making sure there is a 24-hour break from eating, one to three times per week. The only drawback is related to balancing your desire to fast with how you will manage your diabetes.

Clearly when fasting the need for medication and insulin becomes either greatly reduced or much less. Work with your healthcare team, whether it's your doctor, advanced practice clinician, pharmacist, or others, and get their advice on how to manage your medications so you don't have hypoglycemic episodes during this process. Remember, one of your goals may be to get off medication, and fasting will help you achieve that goal. Also keep in mind to arrange your workouts in such a way that you are able to still have a post-workout meal, which is optimal.

20-HOUR FAST (A.K.A WARRIOR DIET)

Do you like the idea of the 24-hour fast but still find yourself a little hungry for a snack two or three hours after dinner? If this sounds like you, then the Warrior Diet may be the perfect fasting solution. The extra time can really provide a less rigid approach to fasting. This approach allows you to fast for 20 hours instead of 24, with the added benefit of a four-hour window to eat. Apparently this is what warriors in various cultures did in the past, hence the name. This is a practical approach to fasting which for many people can be easily incorporated into a healthy lifestyle. Other than trying to get enough healthy calories when you do eat, you will find this type of fasting one of the easiest to follow. Keep in mind, as is the case with the 16/8 Fast, it's okay to take a break over the weekend.

THE 5:2 DIET

With this approach to fasting you simply reduce your calorie consumption on two non-consecutive days of the week, only eating 500 to 600 calories on those days. You follow your normal eating pattern on the other five days. I find this approach more challenging, but have patients who claim it works for them. So experiment and see what works for you.

How Fasting is More Effective at Burning Fat

Now that you have some idea of which fasting options you can consider, let's better understand why I am recommending this as an important approach to helping you fix your diabetes. But keep in mind, no matter which fasting approach you choose, make sure it's simple and sustainable. Why? Because it's the fastest way to quickly burn the fat in your body.

When you eat, you increase insulin production, resulting in the storage of glucose. In your liver and muscle this takes the form of glycogen. In the rest of your body it's fat. When you fast, your insulin production is reduced and you get energy from your glycogen stores first. When these are depleted, energy is taken from the fat in your body. Fasting is more effective than simple calorie reduction because before you start to actually burn fat, you must first deplete your free glucose and glycogen stores, which may take six to eight hours of fasting. In order to start using your fat as an energy source, fasting is needed to deplete your glycogen and free glucose energy sources first, forcing your body to use fat as an energy source.

With this information as your foundation for change, you can now use fasting along with the other dietary recommendations in this book to reduce your calorie consumption, raise your metabolic rate, and better control your blood glucose levels. Fasting is free, simple, and easy to implement. So let's take some lessons from the caveman ancestors who had no choice but to fast often, and return to the hunt-eat-starve approach. This will give your body time to recover from the many metabolic processes that occur while we are eating.

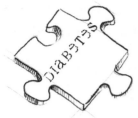

TAKEAWAYS

- Fasting results in the depletion of glycogen and glucose, which results in burning fat as a source of energy.

- Fasting results in the depletion of glycogen and glucose, which results in burning fat as a source of energy.

- Review the four types of intermittent fasting.

- Determine which fasting method fits your lifestyle.

- Make fasting a part of your lifestyle.

CHAPTER 5

Fix Your Knowledge of Diabetic Complications

"A hero is an ordinary individual who finds the strength to persevere and endure in spite of overwhelming obstacles."
~Christopher Reeve

It's About a Lady

One of the biggest heroes I have met was my wife's great-grandmother, Janie. I still remember taking a trip to Port Gibson, Mississippi, while visiting my wife's family and meeting Janie. She was quite the personality. Always greeting me with a smile, she was someone I will never forget. She was also quite the flirt, winking at me every chance she got. I was tempted to warn my wife that she had some competition, but spared her the troubling news. The truth is I was fascinated by Grandma Janie's past. She spent most of her life providing community service to the people of Port Gibson both in her church and as a midwife. In those times, many African-Americans who gave birth did so not with the help of local doctors, but attended by the dedicated midwifes of the community, and Grandma Janie had this special role for Port Gibson.

When my wife reflected on her great-grandmother, she talked about how most of her teachers and other members of the community were delivered by Grandma Janie and regularly gave thanks for her contribution to helping them into this world. And that thanks would be well-earned, since her payment from many of her patients was in the form of chickens, hogs, and other non-monetary means.

Her service to the Port Gibson community was so well regarded that the tools of her trade are now in one of Port Gibson, Mississippi's historical museums. She was truly a gift.

You may have already guessed why I have included Janie in my chapter about diabetic complications. Grandma Janie was diabetic and suffered some of the complications of this condition. If you have a Grandma Janie or want to live as long as she did, avoiding the many complications of diabetics should be one of your goals. The most obvious for Grandma Janie was a leg amputation. When I first met her, she was resting in her bed with her amputated leg stump exposed. At the time of this visit, I was only a college student at Xavier University in Louisiana and did not make the connection between diabetes and amputations. She may have had other complications I was not aware of, but one thing is for sure, diabetes can have a profound effect on one's quality of life.

Grandma Janie will forever be one of my motivations for helping spread knowledge about diabetes and the negative effect it can have on patients and their families and friends. So let's learn a little about these complications so you understand fully why you must fight diabetes. I will start from the head and work my way down to the feet.

Diabetic Complications

BRAIN

What is the most important organ in the body? The brain, heart, lungs, or another? In reality, all organs play critical roles, but the brain literally controls all the others, making it the key. The brain carries out many very important functions, including receiving information from the rest of the body, interpreting that information, and then guiding the body's response to it. The brain also has the job of interpreting odors, light, sounds, and pain. The brain's work does not end there; it also helps perform vital operations such as breathing, maintaining blood pressure, and releasing hormones. Since the brain carries so much responsibility, we must do everything possible to protect it.Diabetes has been linked to an impaired ability to regulate blood flow in the brain. This is likely due to the inflammation that is caused by diabetes. The process of distributing blood as needed to areas of increased neural activity is impaired in diabetics. So when you need extra oxygen the most, during times of increased mental activity, diabetics may not be getting the oxygen they need. This can result in mental and functional decline, based on a study done by Dr. Vera Novak at Harvard Medical School. In minimizing fluctuations of blood sugar levels, inflammation is also minimized, helping to decrease any cognitive decline caused by diabetes.

STROKE

When diabetes is uncontrolled, too much glucose is floating around in your blood. This can lead to increased fatty deposits or clots in your blood vessel walls. Over time this results in decreased blood getting to your brain, ultimately leading to a stroke. In fact, diabetics are 50% more likely than the general population to have a stroke. Once a stroke occurs, the negative effects can be both physical and emotional. Whether it's movement problems, pain, numbness, limited ability to speak, depression, or other known effects, avoiding a stroke should be a top priority.

EYES

Many of us are familiar with the fact that diabetes can lead to blindness. As is the case with stroke, it's all about the blood vessels. When blood glucose levels are elevated, the blood vessels in your eyes are damaged, leading to thickening and leakage. This compromises circulation in the eyes. In some cases, your body will make new, fragile blood vessels, which are prone to leakage. Over time, injured blood vessels can lead to blindness as well as to increased risk of both glaucoma and cataracts.

This is why your doctor may insist you see an ophthalmologist at least every two years if your eyes are healthy and more frequently if they are not. These conditions can be treated, and I've learned over my years of practice that the best treatment is prevention.

GLAUCOMA

When the pressure in your eye rises beyond the normal range of 12-22 mm Hg, glaucoma, or ocular hypertension, could result. Diabetes increases the risk for glaucoma by more than 40 percent. What's the outcome of this high pressure? It leads to pinching of the blood vessels that carry blood to the retina and optic nerve in your eyes. This leads to a gradual loss of vision because the retina and nerve in the eye are damaged.

CATARACTS

Imagine driving your car with a cloudy windshield. It would be difficult at best to make it to your destination. Well, the windshield of your eye is the lens, and if the lens gets cloudy, you essentially have a cataract. When this occurs, the ability to get light through your eyes onto the back of the eye where the retina is becomes compromised, resulting in poor vision. Diabetes increases your risk of cataracts by 60 percent. The good news is that if cataracts become too developed, just like a cloudy windshield, we have the technology to replace it. I hope you will do all you can to keep the lens you were born with.

RETINOPATHY

Uncontrolled diabetes leads to damage of small blood vessels in the eye, resulting in the formation of fragile new blood vessels. The fragility of the new vessels over time will result in bleeding, which in turn will cause cloudy vision and retina damage. If diagnosed early, however, there is time to treat this condition with laser procedures or other procedures like vitrectomy. Either way, regular visits to the eye doctor and controlling your diabetes well remain the mainstays of prevention.

EARS

Not commonly discussed, loss of hearing is twice as likely in diabetics. So many seniors have hearing loss that distinguishing whether their risk was related to diabetes or loud music in the past is hard to determine. What I do know is that hearing loss has a dramatic impact on one's quality of life and preserving your hearing is very important.

MOUTH

Periodontal disease affects one out of five diabetics. By simply having better control of your blood glucose values and visiting the dentist twice per year, you put the odds back in your favor.

HEART

High Blood Pressure:
As discussed previously, uncontrolled diabetes can lead to damage to the walls of your arteries, leading to atherosclerosis. Think of atherosclerotic plaques as being similar to having rust in your water pipes in your home. These plaques reduce the elasticity (flexibility) of your arteries, restricting their ability to expand and ultimately resulting in a higher pressure. Not only does diabetes cause elevated blood pressure, but the resulting elevated blood pressure will increase your risk for heart attacks, strokes, eye problems, and kidney disease. It's a vicious cycle of one problem compounding another. Hypertension is truly a silent killer that we all need to keep under control.

KIDNEYS

Uncontrolled diabetes can damage the kidneys and leave them unable to properly filter the waste from your body. In fact, damage to the kidneys will result in leakage of valuable protein from your body into your urine. This is why your urine protein (micro-albumin test) is checked regularly by your doctor.

High urine protein can be the first signal that something is wrong with the kidneys. This protein warns us that the kidneys are weakening. Dialysis may be the most feared complication of diabetes. This fear is not to be taken lightly, since the outcome of patients with kidney failure is troubling.

A recent study in *Up To Date* reported the following: "once dialysis is started, the range of the expected remaining lifespan in the United States Renal Data System (USRDS) report was approximately eight years (varies with race) for dialysis patients 40 to 44 years of age and approximately 4.5 years for those 60 to 64 years of age."[20]

These realities can be scary for dialysis patients, which is why preventing the need for dialysis is extremely important. Keep in mind that the purpose of mentioning these statistics is not to discourage anyone from using dialysis as a life-saving treatment, but to encourage prevention. For those who need it, dialysis is life-saving.

The good news is that most people with diabetes will never develop kidney disease. The key is to simply take lessons learned about how to control your diabetes and blood pressure, and keep the control in your hands.

STOMACH

Many of my diabetic patients are surprised to learn that even their stomachs can be negatively affected by diabetes. Yes, your stomach. A condition called *gastroparesis* can develop when uncontrolled diabetics have damage to the nerves of their stomachs. As with many of the other conditions discussed in this section, high blood glucose causes chemical changes in the blood vessels, which ultimately compromises the delivery of nutrients to the nerves. This results in nerve damage. The damage to stomach nerves causes delays in how fast stomach contents are emptied. This leads to the many symptoms of gastroparesis, including nausea, vomiting, heartburn, feelings of fullness, abdominal bloating, lack of appetite, painful stomach spasms, and weight loss. I have seen patients with this condition go in and out of the hospital because of either the pain or the inability to keep their food down. This is a not-so-well-known complication that I hope none of my diabetic patients or readers will have to suffer with.

BLADDER

Imagine not having a functional bladder. How would your life be different if you lost control of your bladder because the nerves were damaged by diabetes? This is the life of many diabetics who have lost the ability to control their urine and one of the negative effects of uncontrolled diabetes.

SEXUAL ORGANS

For many of my patients this is the greatest motivation of all. Men have known for some time that diabetes can have an effect on their sexual function. Since it is an uncomfortable subject, sexual issues are often the last thing my male patients bring up an office visit—but rarely is it forgotten. Unfortunately, the same is not true for women. Although many women don't know it, the vaginal dryness they experience may not be menopause, but rather the effects of uncontrolled diabetes and the damage to the nerves of the glands serving the sexual organs. When vaginal nerves don't function properly, vaginal dryness can occur, making sexual intercourse painful.

LEGS

Peripheral arterial disease (PAD) is a condition that affects as many as one in three diabetics over the age of 50. This condition should come as no surprise, since almost every condition we have discussed so far results from the poor circulation that develops when diabetes is not controlled. Narrowing of the arteries in the legs causes this painful condition, limiting the ability of those who suffer from it to walk very far without developing pain. If you experience pain after walking, which is relieved with rest, ask your doctor to evaluate you for this condition.

FEET

Peripheral neuropathy is the result of narrowing of the blood vessels supplying oxygen to the nerves, which leads to nerve dysfunction.

When this nerve damage occurs, you could lose sensation in your feet, leading to a condition called diabetic neuropathy. This could result in sensations of tingling, pain, burning, stabbing, or shooting pains in your feet. The best way to prevent this condition is by controlling your blood glucose values and reversing insulin resistance. This condition is the main reason your doctor should be checking your feet on a regular basis. If your doctor isn't already doing this, take off your shoes before your doctor enters and ask him or her to check your feet.

AUTONOMIC NEUROPATHY

This is the part of the nervous system that controls your bladder, intestinal tract, and sexual organs. So what happens when your bladder nerves are not working? The main problem is that the urine stays in your bladder, increasing the risk of an infection. How about the nerves that go to your sexual organs? If they are affected, erectile dysfunction could occur, which can cause a lot of stress in your marriage or personal life. Even with the knowledge that diabetes is causing this problem, many of my patients still find that their lives are negatively affected by ED, especially if their relationship is volatile or lacking in communication. The intestinal tract can also be affected due to damage to the enteric nerves supplying the small intestine. This can lead to abnormal motility, secretion, or absorption. This can lead to symptoms such as central abdominal pain, bloating, and diarrhea. Furthermore, delayed emptying of fluids in the small intestine may lead to bacterial overgrowth syndromes, resulting in diarrhea and abdominal pain.

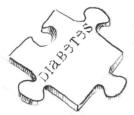

TAKEAWAYS

- Taking control of your diabetes includes knowing how it can affect your body.

- Reducing insulin resistance will help you prevent many of the complications of diabetes.

- Use your newly found knowledge to help encourage self-directed behavioral changes that will improve your overall health and the management of your diabetes.

CHAPTER 6

FIX YOUR UNDERSTANDING OF THE GLYCEMIC INDEX (GI)

*"Disease does not occur unexpectedly; it is the result of constant
violation of Nature's laws. Spreading and accumulation of such
violations transpire suddenly in the form of a disease—
but it only seems sudden."*
~Hippocrates

You've probably either heard about, considered, or tried a low glycemic index approach to eating. It's been a popular diet, especially
for those wanting to lose weight or better control their diabetes.
But staying motivated to stick with the dietary changes can be a
lot to overcome when the rest of the world is not making the same
changes. Although this approach to eating has come in and out of
favor, I wanted to reintroduce the GI concept because I feel it could
be one of many valuable tools to help you make better decisions
about which foods you eat.

Let's be clear. I do not believe in diets of any type. I prefer promoting the idea of replacing one choice over the other. Those choices
are rooted in what your particular goals are and how you respond
to those food choices. Everyone responds to food differently. I have
patients who eat apples with minimal effects on their blood glucose,
while others find apples raise their blood glucose significantly. Your
body will provide all the answers. The purpose of a low glycemic approach is not to follow a strict diet, but to become aware of foods that
are more or less likely to affect your blood glucose values.

The goal is to find the best foods to help you better control your blood glucose. That's why knowing as much as possible about which foods convert to glucose the fastest in your body will be valuable as you work towards the healthiest diet for you.

Cultural and ethnic preferences also affect our food choices. Find foods that align with your particular preference so that your transition from one food choice to another is made as seamlessly as possible. Again, I don't think diets are the answer. But they can sometimes serve as a short-term catalyst that gets us moving in the right direction.

What is the Glycemic Index and the Glycemic Load, and Who Did the Research?

It all started with a Canadian researcher. Once it was discovered that starchy complex carbohydrates can raise sugars as much as table sugar does, this researcher, Dr. David Jenkins, proposed the idea of the glycemic index in 1981. Then in 1997, research done at Harvard proposed that a concept called the glycemic load could account for differences in the carbohydrate content in meals. The University of Sydney, however, has been responsible for the bulk of the research needed to help us determine which foods are helping or hurting us. Their website, www.glycemicindex.com, should be considered the standard for identifying foods with a high or low glycemic index.

This website defines the glycemic index in the following way: "The glycemic index (GI) is a ranking of carbohydrates on a scale from 0 to 100 according to the extent to which they raise blood sugar levels after eating. Foods with a high GI are those which are rapidly digested and absorbed and result in marked fluctuations in blood sugar levels. Low-GI foods, by virtue of their slow digestion and absorption, produce gradual rises in blood sugar and insulin levels, and have proven benefits for health. Low GI diets have been shown to improve both glucose and lipid levels in people with diabetes (Type 1 and Type 2). They have benefits for weight control because they help control appetite and delay hunger. Low GI diets also reduce insulin levels and insulin resistance." [21]

As you can see, this research provided evidence that eating low glycemic index foods would help diabetics as well as help those trying to lose weight or improve their cholesterol levels. The website also shares the following: "Recent studies from Harvard School of Public Health indicate that the risks of diseases such as Type 2 diabetes and coronary heart disease are strongly related to the GI of the overall diet. In 1999, the World Health Organization (WHO) and Food and Agriculture Organization (FAO) recommended that people in industrialized countries base their diets on low-GI foods in order to prevent the most common diseases of affluence, such as coronary heart disease, diabetes and obesity." [22]

Examples of Low, Medium, and High GI Foods

Now that you have an idea where the glycemic index came from, let's look at some examples of foods that are categorized as low, medium, or high GI foods. The following lists are from the American Diabetes Association website.

LOW GI FOODS (55 OR LESS)

- 100 percent stone-ground whole wheat or pumpernickel bread

- Oatmeal (rolled or steel-cut), oat bran, muesli

- Pasta, converted rice, barley, bulgar

- Sweet potato, corn, yam, lima/butter beans, peas, legumes, and lentils

- Most fruits, non-starchy vegetables, and carrots

MEDIUM GI FOODS (56-69)

- Whole wheat, rye, and pita bread

- Quick oats

- Brown, wild, or basmati rice; couscous

HIGH GI FOODS (70 OR MORE)

- White bread or bagel

- Corn flakes, puffed rice, bran flakes, instant oatmeal

- Short-grain white rice, rice pasta, macaroni-and-cheese from mix

- Russet potato, pumpkin

- Pretzels, rice cakes, popcorn, saltine crackers

- Melons and pineapple [24]

Food with a high GI raises blood glucose more than food with a medium or low GI. So your overall goal is to look at what you are currently eating to determine where there may be some room for exchanging higher GI foods for lower GI foods. This can be a challenge, depending on your eating habits.

For example, I attended Xavier University of Louisiana for undergraduate studies and ate a lot of red beans and rice while in school. I would never ask someone from New Orleans to stop eating rice because its glycemic index is high. I would, however, suggest switching to a lower glycemic version of rice. For example, Uncle Ben's rice has a lower glycemic index than other brands.

Even better is using cauliflower as a rice alternative. By simply using a cheese grater or food processor, cauliflower can be easily converted to a rice alternative. Even more amazing is the fact that a serving of cauliflower rice may only yield four to five carbs, whereas the same serving of white or brown rice yields 40 to 45 carbs. That's ten times as many carbs. It is certainly worth it to at least give this alternative a chance. It could be life-altering for anyone who regularly uses rice as a foundation of their diet.

Another strategy is to combine high GI foods with low GI foods. This can help balance the meal. For example, let's revisit my red beans and rice days. Combining the rice with red beans helps lighten the effect of high-carb rice. Take a look at the glycemic index of the following options:

- Quick cook white rice: GI 67

- Brown rice: GI 50

- Uncle Ben's White rice: GI 38

- Red beans: GI 29

As you can see, red beans have a low glycemic index. They contain a lot of fiber, which slows down the digestion of the carb, resulting in a slower rise in your blood glucose values. So if the idea of cauliflower rice with your beans can't be adjusted to in your home, make sure to add beans to your rice so that you eat your rice with minimal harm to your diabetes goals.

You must take manageable and practical steps when making your changes. I know you may not be feeding just yourself, so keeping the needs of your household in perspective is sometimes needed. But remember, it's not about them, it's about you. Don't compromise your health trying to keep everyone else happy. You are becoming the expert on nutrition. By sharing what you've learned, you could convince others to join you on this food journey. And the best thing you could do? Presenting them with delicious food alternatives. That will sell it better than anything.

What Affects the GI of a Food?

Thankfully, the glycemic index of a food is affected by factors other than fiber content. It reminds me of how our environment affects how we act or what we become. I tell my kids, who you hang with matters and may have as big an impact on who you become as anything you do in your lifetime. My own personal story provides a good example of this. When I was in New Orleans, enjoying that good Cajun and creole food, my first semester as a student was my weakest. As much as I enjoyed the friends I spent time with, my overall performance was similar to many of the students that struggled. I soon recognized I was not laying the foundation needed for a medical school applicant. But something magical happened when I started studying and hanging out with one of our school's strongest students, Dobbin Bookman, now a leader at Harvard. I soon learned through him how to be a great student and became one of the school's strongest students as well. I did this by mirroring his study habits, which resulted in the development of great study habits. The habits of my newly found friend, who still remains a source of advice and counsel, was the catalyst I needed to get back on track. I am forever grateful for this relationship, which helped me understand how important it is to surround yourself with people who help make you better. So remember, think long and hard about who you hang out with. It could be a matter of your success or failure.

This is also true of your food. Which foods are you hanging out with? Are they making you healthier? Are they serving you in a positive way or one that is harmful to your body? Foods with a lower glycemic index are like my college study buddy—they can help you fix your diabetes. It's time to do an inventory to see if you are "keeping good company." It's time to rid yourself of foods that are not allowing you to be your very best. Foods with a low glycemic index are the ones that are more likely to get you to your goals. All you need to do is the research to discover which ones you need to add to your plate.

Glycemic Index Factors that Cause Variation

Imagine spending the next year eating what you felt was a food with a low glycemic index, only to find out that you did not consume it in the lowest glycemic state. You'd be frustrated and more likely to give up. To prevent this, I want to make sure you acquire some basic understanding of what factors can affect the GI of the foods you eat. Let's take a look at some of those factors.

RIPENESS

The ripeness of a food will definitely affect the GI of many fruits and vegetables. A ripe banana may have a GI of 52, while an underripe banana could have a GI as low as 30. Although both values are good, using the lower GI option may be the better decision. You may not even notice the difference when you are putting a less-ripe banana in your smoothie.

COMBINATIONS

Yes! What you combine with your higher carb foods could make all the difference in the world. If you think about it, your body is not worried about how the food gets into you. The only thing your digestive system knows is that it has to do the work of digestion. Although the digestive process will be different depending on the food that is being processed, all foods impact each other as the process is occurring. As an example, if healthy fat-rich avocado is added to a fruit smoothie, the overall glycemic index of the drink will be reduced. The avocado takes longer for your body to process, so glucose takes longer to enter your cells. Combining lower glycemic foods with higher GI foods can minimize the sugar spikes. You need to keep your blood sugars at the right level as often as possible. Of course, how foods interact with each other varies, but combining foods with high and low GI is a good rule to live by.

PROCESSING

The process of transforming a raw ingredient, by physical or chemical means, into food can have a significant effect on its glycemic index. A good example of this is potatoes, one of the most popular carbohydrates in the world.

How quickly potato starch is broken down depends on many factors, including the variety of the potato, the age, and the processing technique, such as boiling, baking, microwaving, roasting, or frying.

Research reported in *Food Research International* revealed that french-fried potatoes contain more resistant starch, whereas boiled and mashed potatoes are less resistant. In other words, they found that french-fried potatoes don't impact your blood glucose as much as boiled or mashed potatoes. This is combined with the fact that, cooling or storing of french-fried potatoes, after processing significantly reduces the GI due to retrogradation of starch molecules.[25] This was surprising to me as much as it may be to you. I am not suggesting that you eat french fries because they are more resistant; I just want you to understand the concept that some forms of white potatoes have less of a carb impact.

COOKING METHOD

How you prepare your food will either raise or lower the glycemic index. Cooking makes dietary carbohydrates more available to digestive enzymes and raises the glycemic index. Any cooking method that breaks apart a grain or adds heat to a grain or carbohydrate will raise the GI. According to Harvard Medical School, carrots have a glycemic index ranking of 47, plus or minus 16. The number depends on a number of factors but in general, cooked carrots have a higher GI than raw carrots. Juiced carrots have an even higher GI for the reasons I just described: less fiber.

ADDING FAT OR FIBER

I know I keep drumming this issue into your head, but I plan to keep on doing it. Adding fat or fiber will slow down carbohydrate digestion and absorption, lowering the GI. For example, cooking food in oils, as opposed to boiling in water, lowers the GI. This explains why fried french fries have a lower GI than baked potatoes. Even using a microwave or boiling will raise the GI versus baking or steaming. The more aggressive the cooking method at breaking down the foods, the more likely that process will raise the GI.

Fiber, like fat, has an effect on the glycemic index of food. But not all fibers are the same. Fiber found in whole wheat, for example, is insoluble and has little effect on the glycemic index. Soluble fiber, on the other hand, lowers the glycemic index. Foods high in soluble fiber, such as oats, barley, and legumes (dried beans and lentils), have low glycemic index values.

VARIETY

I know it seems odd that the shape of a food will affect its glycemic index. But research suggests the end result, as it relates to GI, will be different. For example, long-grain white rice has a lower GI than short-grain rice. So whenever you decide to eat this higher-carb food, make sure you use the long-grain version. This is a good point to mention that you don't want to take yourself too seriously. It's okay to have a cheat day periodically and indulge in those so called "comfort foods" you have enjoyed over the years.

Why Spikes in Your Blood Sugars Can Make You Sick

When high GI foods are ingested, elevation in glucose occurs, which leads to an increase in insulin production. Believe it or not, this leads to inflammation which negatively effects endothelial (blood vessel cell wall) function. You can only imagine what happens when cell walls become inflamed. Those arteries develop plaques (atherosclerosis) and subsequently increased risk of clots (thrombotic disease).

Ultimately, the high insulin production puts stress on the beta cells in the pancreas, so that they eventually become overworked, which leads to diabetes. So give your pancreas a break. Eat more foods that don't require it to work overtime.

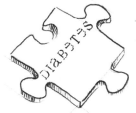

TAKEAWAYS

- Diets don't work. Learning how to make better food choices does.

- Having multiple meals with low glycemic indexes will put less stress on the beta cells in your pancreas.

- Pay more attention to the quality of your food and less to the quantity.

- Help curb hunger by drinking plenty of water.

- Surround yourself with people who will keep you motivated (remember the story of my college friend).

- Stop taking yourself too seriously and cheat periodically.

- It's about doing what's best for you and no one else. It's time to be a little selfish.

CHAPTER 7

FIX YOUR FEAR OF FATS

"I like food. I like eating.
And I don't want to deprive myself of good food."
~Sarah Michelle Gellar

Fix Your FEAR of FATs

I did something truly amazing. I got a cable/Internet bill that exceeded $270 for the month. My frustration with that bill led me to "cut the cord" and get rid of cable permanently. That was a great decision with unexpected consequences. One was that I have a lot more time to do more important things than watch television. It saved my family $200/month that we now invest in the children's futures. The other $70 pays for the Internet connection. Cutting off cable television also reduced my exposure to constant headlines reminding me of the latest recommendations of what to add to or remove from my diet. It's hard to know what to do with so much contradictory information. Years of exposure to all this clutter on television has led to many of the beliefs I have about food, including the following:

• Processed Low-Fat Foods Are Healthy Options

• Eating Fat Makes You Fat and High-Fat Diets Are Dangerous

• A Low-Fat, High-Carb Diet is the Optimal Diet

I could list others, but the real question is, are these claims true? Instead of addressing each one, let's take a look at diabetes and its relationship to the carbohydrates, fats, and proteins in our diet.

Let's start with carbs. You've already learned that most people with Type 2 diabetes have a resistance to insulin. You also know that insulin simply wants to do its job and move glucose from your blood into your cells. The problem occurs when we ask our insulin-producing cells in the pancreas to make more insulin than is reasonable, resulting in a pancreas that cranks out more and more insulin. Imagine having to do this over and over again with each meal. What are the chances your pancreas will become fatigued? This may not happen right away. Like most organs in the body, the pancreas can keep up with most of the body's demands. But over time the insulin-producing beta cells will become overworked and lose much of their ability to keep up with the demands of high-carb eating. This is called hyperinsulinemia.

Hyperinsulinemia also greatly increases our risk for developing other diseases, including cardiovascular disease, obesity, metabolic syndrome, and other endocrine disorders.

Avoiding hyperinsulinemia cannot be done by taking more and more medicine, but by reducing the amount of carbohydrates we ask our pancreas to process with each meal. Combining a low-carb diet with increased physical activity is a simple yet effective way to avoid hyperinsulinemia.

In addition to its role in regulating glucose metabolism, insulin stimulates lipogenesis, diminishes lipolysis, and increases amino acid transport into cells. That's a little scientific, so let's break it down. Lipogenesis is the process of making fat, and lipolysis is the breakdown of fat. You don't have to be a rocket scientist to know that making more fat and reserving it is not something you want unless you are a bear preparing for hibernation. Therefore, anything we can do to decrease the need for all that insulin should be a priority.

Finally, glucose levels must be in balance to prevent the high spikes in blood glucose commonly seen in high glycemic index diets. Eating low glycemic index foods enables you to avoid those blood-glucose spikes and in turn avoid insulin surges. This is important because surges usually result in cravings for more food. You then need more insulin to deal with the glucose you just ingested, and the cycle continues. So if you want to avoid cravings and blood glucose spikes, consider eating foods that don't cause spikes, like fats or low glycemic index foods. Let's stop using medicines to fix what our diet can do much more effectively.

Let's take a look at the current recommendations from the ADA on carbohydrate ingestion:

- Ingest moderate carbohydrate level (about 45 percent of calories come from carbohydrates).

- Carbohydrate intake is spread throughout the day.

- Most meals have 45 to 60 grams of carbohydrate.

- Most snacks have 10 to 25 grams of carbohydrate.

- Limit trans fats as much as possible, <10 percent of calories from saturated fat, and focus on healthy or «good» fat sources.[29]

Now before I say anything else, you should know that the American Diabetes Association is an organization I speak on behalf of and fully support. They have been the leaders in diabetes education, leading the fight against the deadly consequences of diabetes and providing support for all who face it. They also fund research to prevent, cure, and manage diabetes, while also delivering vital services to hundreds of communities. Having said that, it seems to me that some of the recommendations are counter-productive, considering the fact that I have suggested a low-carbohydrate diet is the way to go. The reality is that there remains much controversy about which way to approach diabetes treatment, and the ADA makes the best recommendation based on the available science. The take-home message for me, however, would be to be open to carbs with a lower glycemic index and fats that are healthier. By combining both concepts, we may be able to create dietary approaches that get us to the goal of reducing blood glucose spikes.

Much of the research that supports my recommendations requires a new approach, focusing on the *cause* of Type 2 diabetes (insulin resistance) and not the *symptoms* (high blood glucose). Once organizations also incorporate this research and change their focus, we will all be aligned in our message. And that is reducing the need for medication by teaching that a low-carb and high-healthy-fat diet, with few processed foods, is the best approach for fixing diabetes.

Now you may ask, will reducing carbohydrates put me at risk? Don't I need carbohydrates to live? Will I become carbohydrate deficient if I avoid carbs? While exploring the risks and benefits of carbohydrate restriction, I was surprised to find little evidence that exogenous carbohydrate is needed for human function. The American Journal of Clinical Nutrition stated there is no minimum requirement or essential requirements for carbs.

The currently established human essential nutrients are water, energy, amino acids (histidine, isoleucine, leucine, lysine, methionine, phenylalanine, threonine, tryptophan, and valine), essential fatty acids (linoleic and α-linolenic acids), vitamins (ascorbic acid, vitamin A, vitamin D, vitamin E, vitamin K, thiamine, riboflavin, niacin, vitamin B-6, pantothenic acid, folic acid, biotin, and vitamin B-12), minerals (calcium, phosphorus, magnesium, and iron), trace minerals (zinc, copper, manganese, iodine, selenium, molybdenum, and chromium), electrolytes (sodium, potassium, and chloride), and ultratrace minerals.[30]

Note the absence of specific carbohydrates from this list.

I am not suggesting that it would make any rational sense not to eat carbs at all. I am simply stating that reducing the carbs in your diet is not likely to cause you harm. The main message here is that the diet I am advocating is not high protein, or zero carbohydrate. It is a diet where healthier fats as well as high quality low glycemic index carbs and protein are the focus.

Fat has less effect on your blood glucose levels than any other component of your diet.[28] Proteins are in second place, while carbohydrates have the greatest effect. As a result, the insulin spikes you are attempting to avoid are easier to manage if you simply increase the amount of fat you consume in your diet.

Now that you better understand why FAT is not bad, you have the basic foundation and confidence you need to start adding healthy fats to your diet. So the next time you make a healthy smoothie or are planning your dinner, don't forget to incorporate the healthy fats into your list of ingredients.

Things to Consider as You Make Changes to Your Diet

I want you to view your food choices not as what you **can't** eat but rather what you **can**, specifically the new foods you are adding to your diet. So instead of thinking about the carbs you can't eat, think about the ones you are replacing them with. For example, when we wanted to cut back on pasta in our home, we switched from our usual starchy spaghetti to zucchini pasta made by using a zucchini splicer. Initially, I expected my family to push back, but it turned out they found the zucchini spaghetti to be just as enjoyable. The process of replacing was very effective and simple.

So how do you enjoy a low-carb, high-fat diet without eating primarily meat? There is so much controversy around high-fat diets that most doctors struggle to recommend them even if the research around this concept is more supportive. We were taught low fat, high fiber in our medical training. Low-carb, high-fat is the opposite of what we've been taught for years. To overcome this, simply add fat in the most healthy way possible. Take lessons from our vegetarian friends by focusing on the fats in plants like the avocado.

Eating a low-carb diet while attempting to eliminate or reduce meat seems challenging, but as you will see, it's possible once you know how to select the right foods. One of the main concerns I've heard from my patients is that starchy foods like potatoes are very filling and eating less of them could lead to feeling hungry. The reality is that research supports the idea that eating a diet with less carbs and more fat could actually reduce appetite, allowing you to eat fewer calories.[31, 32] Another concern I hear often is that low-carb diets may be harmful to your cholesterol. Again, research doesn't bear this out. In fact, research has revealed that this type of diet reduces triglycerides, raises HDL (the "good") cholesterol, and lowers blood pressure. You may ask, "Who benefits the most from eating a higher fat diet?" The answer is simply, your average diabetic.

Now that I have primed you, let's look at some of the healthy fats you can now start reintroducing back into your diet.

EGGS

Eggs are one of the best sources of fat and protein. Most of us have been told at some point that eating eggs could be harmful because they increase the risk of heart disease. It just seems reasonable that egg yolks, which contain a high amount of cholesterol, would be harmful to us. Research on this topic, however, suggests that for most of the population, there is at best a small effect on our blood levels of total cholesterol and the harmful LDL cholesterol. In fact, one egg per day does not increase the risk of heart disease in healthy individuals.[33, 34]

Because diabetes does increase risk for heart disease, however, egg whites may be a better option. If egg yolks are ingested, limiting the amount to two or three per week is best.[35] The best approach may be to compare your cholesterol before and after increasing your whole egg consumption. If you find your cholesterol is unaffected by the increased consumption, you may consider continuing consumption of whole eggs. Only 15 percent of the population is negatively affected by consuming whole eggs.

AVOCADOS

Growing up, I never had any exposure to avocados and when I finally did, its green appearance did not seem particularly attractive. As my diet changed, however, I was willing to consider it and tried it initially as guacamole. When prepared with the right additions, guacamole can be very tasty and has become one of my favorite fruits. In fact, our local grocer offers it already prepared and we buy it almost every week. It offers a great after-school/work snack or can be eaten during the lunch hour. Unlike most fruit, which tends not to be fatty, this fruit is filled with healthy fats (77 percent of its calories). Avocados are also rich in potassium, are a great source of fiber, and have positive effects on our cholesterol.

CHEESE

I'm not sure whether my recommendation of eggs or cheese is more surprising, but the research supports including cheese in our diets. It's an excellent source of protein; it's rich in calcium and good bacteria; and it contains healthy fatty acids with the capacity to actually reduce Type 2 diabetes risks.

With its great taste and nutritional benefits, cheese is one of the easiest foods to add to a balanced diet with minimal effects on blood glucose levels.

FATTY FISH

The benefits of fatty fish are many and that's why the American Heart Association recommends eating fish (particularly fatty fish) at least two times (two servings) a week. Why? Because fish is a good source of omega-3 fatty acids, which decreases the risk for heart-related conditions like abnormal heartbeats (arrhythmias), which could lead to sudden death. It also decreases triglyceride levels, lowers blood pressure, and decreases the growth rate of atherosclerotic plaques. Examples of fatty fish include my favorite—salmon—as well as mackerel, herring, lake trout, sardines, and albacore tuna. So as unappealing as the term "fatty fish" may be, start enjoying more of these tasty and healthy foods.

DARK CHOCOLATE

I know what many of you are thinking, you love chocolate but dark chocolate not so much. I can totally relate. When I first gave dark chocolate a try, it tasted bitter. I was only trying it for its health benefits and nothing more. I later developed a taste for it, and dark chocolate has become one of my favorite end-of-the-day snacks. Your palate is used to the sugar-filled chocolate that is prevalent in our society. But I've learned from personal experience that you can retrain your palate. And it's worth it. Dark chocolate has about 65 percent of its calories from fat and contains fiber, iron, magnesium, copper, and antioxidants. People who eat dark chocolate are less likely to die from heart disease.

CHIA SEEDS

The history of chia seeds goes back to 3500 B.C., when the Aztecs used them as one of their main foods. Chia was later used between 1500 and 900 B.C. by people in Mexico to make medicine, ground flour, and oil. The ancient Mayan civilization even believed the seeds possessed supernatural powers, giving them energy. It is still considered a good food to boost your energy levels.

Chia seeds have about 9 grams of fat in each ounce, and a lot of fiber as well. Another great benefit is that the fat within these seeds is primarily the healthy omega-3 fat known for its blood pressure and anti-inflammatory benefits. And I love the chia seeds because they don't really affect the taste of foods much, and my family has no idea that I add them to their foods/smoothies. So the next time you have a smoothie, consider adding some chia seeds to power your smoothie to a whole new level.

NUTS

I write this section with some sadness because I am allergic to tree nuts. Unfortunately, tree nut allergies are very common, and in some cases can cause fatal allergic reactions. But not all nuts are what they seem. For example, I can eat regular peanuts all day long, because they are actually legumes. I can also eat seeds like sunflower and sesame. So when you find a recipe that includes nuts, and you also suffer from tree nut allergies, simply replace the tree nuts with other options you are not allergic to. I don't worry about what I can't have. I focus on what I can. It's a simple life lesson that will help ensure you are a happier person.

Why do we care about adding nuts to our diets? Well, because nuts are loaded with fats, fiber, vitamin E, magnesium, and minerals. They are the perfect between-meal snacks for a diabetic, or anyone wanting to have a healthier diet. Research supports the many benefits of reducing risk of heart disease, obesity, and of course diabetes. So when possible, try adding some of the many varieties of healthy nuts to your diet.

COCONUTS AND COCONUT OIL

Coconuts are not a botanical nut. They are classified as a fruit, even though the Food and Drug Administration recognizes coconut as a tree nut. Of course, there are people with tree nut allergies who may have a reaction to coconuts, so discuss this with an allergist before trying them. The same can be said of nutmeg, which is derived from seeds, not nuts, and is usually consumed without risk. This is trivia for non-tree nut allergic readers, but I hope that for those who have avoided coconuts, it will give you the confidence to research whether this would be a good option for you.

So what are the benefits? Coconuts are a rich source of saturated fat: 90 percent of their fatty acids are saturated. Coconut fatty acids are metabolized differently from other fats, with a direct path to the liver, where they are turned into ketone bodies. Benefits of coconuts include increased metabolic rate, appetite suppression, and ultimately less belly fat.

EXTRA-VIRGIN OLIVE OIL

We've all heard about the benefits of olive oil in cooking. What you might not know is that extra-virgin olive oil has better anti-inflammatory benefits than regular olive oil. Extra-virgin olive oil is considered an unrefined oil since it's not treated with chemicals or altered by temperature. Olive oil's fat is more beneficial because 75 percent of its fat is in the form of oleic acid (a monounsaturated, omega-9 fatty acid). This is higher than other oil options. Research has found that increasing the monounsaturated, omega-9 acid in your diet, results in decreases in total blood cholesterol, LDL cholesterol (bad), and blood pressure. Extra virgin olive oil also contains many vitamins, including vitamins E and K. There is no doubt that of the oil options, extra virgin olive oil is the clear winner. So enjoy.

FULL-FAT YOGURT

Once again, I'm going to tell you that fat is not the enemy. Numerous studies show that full-fat dairy in our diet produces smaller waistlines (less belly fat), and reduces the risk of heart disease, as well as diabetes. I know it will be hard to shop for whole milk or full-fat yogurt, but research is telling us to do just that. Besides these benefits, yogurt also provides healthy probiotic bacteria, resulting in improved digestion.

Keep in mind when shopping, however, that most yogurts are loaded with added sugars. Shopping for plain yogurt and adding your own flavor with fruit or vanilla extract is a better way to go.

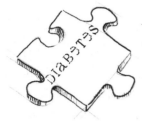

TAKEAWAYS

- High-fat diets helps your body avoid hyperinsulin states, which are inflammatory.

- Lower-carbohydrate diets are safe, since carbs are not an essential nutrient.

- Fat has less effect on your blood glucose levels than any other component of your diet.

- View your food choices not as what you CAN'T eat but rather what you CAN, specifically the new foods you are adding to your diet.

- Start incorporating high-fat foods into your diet.

CHAPTER **8**

Fix Your Smoothies

"Let food be thy medicine and medicine be thy food."
~Hippocrates

Smoothies

The old you might have questioned how a diabetic could drink a smoothie. But the new you knows that different carbohydrates are processed differently by your body, and that by mixing the right food combinations you can create a diabetic-friendly smoothie.

Are you ready to make some dietary changes with that new knowledge? I sure was. But like many of you, my biggest barrier was time. Creating healthy smoothies emerged as the perfect solution.

What I discovered was that if all the necessary items were available, including green vegetables, a liquid base, and fruit, the process of preparing a healthy smoothie would only take about 10 minutes or less most mornings. It became a habit that was easy to duplicate once we got going.

Keep in mind, this is not dieting, it's just an alternative to how the food gets into you. It's a simple way to eat healthier, feel better, and have the energy you need to get through a long day. Why not give your body the nutrients it needs to fight life's stressors?

How Smoothies Can Change Your Life

Once I switched from my daily oatmeal to nutrient-packed smoothies, I received the gift of removing many of the processed foods out of my diet. Yes, even instant oatmeal is overly processed (try steel-cut instead). In fact, most packaged foods are overly processed. I had never really thought about the fact that many of the foods I was eating could be called "dead food," sitting on the supermarket shelf for longer than any of us would like to think about. Each time I shopped for food, I spent too much time walking away from the living food on the outer edges of the grocery store where the fruits and vegetables were found. I started to realize that what you put into your body is exactly what you get out. I also know that natural whole foods are naturally not addictive. In fact, when was the last time you overate the pears or bananas on your counter? It simply doesn't happen. I learned that Mother Nature is not in the business of creating addicts. On the other hand, humankind with its fancy labs and researchers have done a great job creating foods that you will come back for over and over again. Remember this: the food industry is in the business of making money, not keeping you healthy.

After drinking healthy smoothies for some time, I noticed that my energy was not the only aspect of my life that was changing. It seemed I never got sick any more. I realized through experience and research that healthy whole foods were the best preventive medicine. I postulated that my immune system must have become more effective at warding off germs even when they entered my body. This resulted in never missing work due to sick days, which for me is extremely important, since I would have to cancel as many as 30 patient visits for the day if this were to occur. I certainly did not want to do this to my patients and fortunately did not need to. As the quote from Hippocrates that begins this chapter suggests: food is a source of healing that many of us have overlooked. It's time to open our eyes and take the natural medicine the universe has already provided us: food.

Whether your first meal is at breakfast or lunch (I tend to fast for breakfast and have smoothies for lunch), start the day with living food. Acknowledge that what you put into your body is what you will get out of it. If you put life into your body, life will come out of you. If you put death into your body, death will be the outcome. So although you can't really see it right now because your life has become a 24-hour grind, you will soon find the time to incorporate smoothies because your focus will shift. So now that you have some inspiration, let's learn more about smoothie-making so you can start to see how it may fit into your lifestyle.

Benefits of Drinking Smoothies

Smoothies give you a unique opportunity to drink many of the foods that you know are healthy but that are difficult to get into your diet on a regular basis. Just think about how many times you actually ingested kale, spirulina, or chia seeds in the last week. For most of us, it simply would not have happened. Smoothies, on the other hand, provide an easy mechanism for regularly eating all of those healthy foods. Let's review some of the benefits of drinking smoothies.

Convenience: Preparing smoothies may seem like a hassle, especially if you have to get up early for work or because of the noise the blender makes. But the reality is that it only takes me about 10 minutes to prepare my average smoothie. Smoothies have also made my lunch hour more efficient. I usually enjoy my smoothie while working on my patients' electronic charts during the lunch hour. I can't imagine returning to the old routine of waiting for an available microwave to warm up my lunch, or even worse, making a trip to a take-out place in search for lunch. Those days are long gone.

Fiber: So many of my patients complain of digestive irregularity, and what bothers them the most is constipation. The high fiber content of smoothies can help with this. In fact, many who drink smoothies have to adjust to all the fiber in smoothies. This usually resolves over time, so if this is your experience, allow your body to adjust by easing smoothies into your routine.

Affordable: Purchasing green smoothies in a smoothie bar can be expensive, but at home the costs are much more reasonable. In fact, when compared to less healthy options, smoothies can be quite affordable. The hard part is your perception. If you consider a smoothie your meal and compare prices that way, you will find that smoothies are quite reasonable.

Great for weight loss: Since green smoothies are low in calories as well as filling due to high fiber content, they can make you feel full, which helps if you are on the weight loss journey. For many of my patients it's the easiest weight loss plan they have ever tried.

Easy to digest: Your digestive system will appreciate the fact that your blender has done much of the work for it. After all, it has blended the ingredients before they enter your stomach. You use less energy, which can be used for other important bodily functions.

Antioxidants, digestive enzymes, and vitamins: Many of the foods added to smoothies will contain plenty of the antioxidants, vitamins, and enzymes you will need to be healthy. It is hard to imagine an easier way to get so much with so little.

General Principles to Consider for Smoothies

Water: Whenever possible, your liquid base should be water. Juices add unnecessary sugars and calories. Another way to flavor your smoothie without adding juice is to use a scoop of your favorite powder, such as Barlean's organic berry greens. Although the powder does contain a small amount of carbs, it would be a much better alternative than juices.

Stevia: Avoid adding sweeteners to your smoothies as a general rule. Your ultimate goal is to adjust your taste buds to a less sweet taste, fixing that sweet tooth you've developed over time. If sweetness is needed, however, consider stevia as your go-to sweetener. Other options include xylitol or erythritol. Full disclosure: when I consider all the processing needed to convert a plant like stevia to a sweetener (which may include 40 to 90 steps!), I am not convinced that this is any better than using an artificial sweetener.

Fruits: Lower-carb fruits are a great addition to any smoothie. They provide enough taste to mask the flavor of less tasty vegetables, while not adding a high amount of carbs. Berries work great for this purpose, and also provide great health benefits.

Flexibility: You will be asked to try items you either don't currently like or have never eaten before. Changing how you eat will be challenging, but it's worth it. Use the ideas as a foundation, then add your own touches, as long as they comply with the low-carb recommendations. Keep in mind that fat and protein will help curb your appetite, so add more of these ingredients when needed.

The need to chew: Some people simply can't imagine drinking their meals because they are accustomed to the act of chewing. For those people, it may be helpful to chew the nuts or seeds you would have otherwise put in your smoothies. This can be done before, during, or right after enjoying your smoothie.

Important Smoothie Ingredients

STEVIA

Let's begin our discussion about ingredients with some additional comments about stevia. The biggest challenge I faced when I told my family we were going to make our smoothies diabetic-friendly was the knowledge that they needed to contain lower glycemic fruit, which may not be as sweet as their palates were accustomed to. I discovered, however, that the way to help make this transition easier was to add something sweet to the smoothie. That something for my family was stevia.

Most low-calorie sweeteners have a potency much greater than sugar, and stevia is no exception. Many people have asked me how anything can have zero calories. The answer is that with the exception of aspartame, none of the sweeteners can be broken down by the body. They simply go straight through our digestive system. Stevia is a highly purified product that comes from the stevia plant. As with most sweeteners, it's much sweeter than sugar. It has various brand names, including A Sweet Leaf, Sun Crystals, Stevia, Truvia, and PureVia. I like Stevia because it is plant=based and not an artificial product. Again, as mentioned earlier, the ideal state is allowing your palate to adjust to the natural tastes of foods. But if that seems impossible, I'm happy stevia is available as a nice option for diabetics with a sweet tooth.

The high sugar content of many smoothies is what makes many of them less desirable for diabetics, so having low-sugar options will be key to making sure your smoothies don't sabotage your efforts to create a healthy meal replacement.

The following list of ingredients are a sampling of additional food choices that can help you achieve your goal of avoiding a glucose spike when you drink your smoothie.

HEMP SEEDS

This is an excellent source of protein containing 21 known amino acids, nine of which your body can't produce on its own. Two tablespoons of hemp protein powder can provide around 13 to 15 grams of protein, and it's easier for your body to process than other protein sources. This plant-based protein is one of my favorite protein supplements. If you are avoiding dairy (whey protein) or have concerns about too much soy (soy protein), hemp protein can be a great alternative.

AVOCADO

I can't believe I did not discover this nutritious fruit until late in my adulthood. This fruit is one of the most nutritious on the planet, con-taining more than 20 different vitamins and minerals. It also contains protein and fiber, and most important, it's loaded with healthy fats. This is one of the key ingredients for diabetic-friendly smoothies, and even if you historically have not been a fan of avocado, this is one fruit you may want to try again.

Just FYI: the International table of glycemic index and glycemic load values published in 2002 by researchers from the University of Sydney did not include the GI values for avocados because even in large amounts they are not likely to raise blood glucose values.

Keep in mind, when you are faced with a suggestion that initially turns you off, you must be willing to give it a chance. For example, I was never a fan of raw carrots but recognized that they offered many health benefits. So in order to get those benefits, I added raw carrots to my smoothies, which to my surprise made them a little sweeter tasting while also allowing me to reap all those nutritional benefits. With a little creativity, you'll find that there are many ingredients you can add to your smoothie and the taste will be masked by the other ingredients.

CUCUMBER

Cucumbers are something most of us don't eat enough of and they are a great healthy addition to any smoothie. One of the keys to being a successful smoothie creator is the ability to add as many healthy ingredients as possible that don't negatively impact flavor. Cucumbers are perfect for this, since they have a very mild taste. They add zero sugar and a lot of moisture. They also have many vitamins, are anti-inflammatory, and have antioxidant properties as well.

SEED AND NUT BUTTERS

One of the great things about nut and seed butters is that, like cucumbers, they don't change the taste of smoothies much, allowing you to get the benefits without losing flavor. They also make your smoothies creamier, more nutritious, and more filling—preventing you from suffering from cravings. Loaded with monounsaturated fatty acid (MUFA) and polyunsaturated fatty acid (PUFA), they will help lower the risk of heart disease and diabetes. Varieties you can add to your smoothies include peanut butter, almond butter, cashew butter, sunflower seed butter, hemp seed butter, soy butter, and walnut butter. When adding nut butters to your smoothies, don't overdo it initially. You'll notice the texture change, so allow yourself time to adjust.

SOMETHING GREEN LIKE SPINACH

"Make sure to put something green into your smoothies," is what I usually tell my patients when we have conversations about smoothies. Spinach has become my favorite, primarily because it's easy to find, and like some of the other ingredients described so far, it has minimal effect on taste. Spinach is known for its high nutritional content, its ability to restore energy, and for being rich in iron. It's also loaded with vitamins and minerals, including manganese, magnesium, vitamin K, and vitamin B2. Once you get accustomed to adding spinach to your smoothies, it's time to open up the possibilities and try other green items like kale, broccoli, and green cabbage. The options are endless.

CINNAMON

Why cinnamon? Research has shown that cinnamon supplements can lower blood glucose levels in people with Type 2 diabetes. Besides this obvious benefit, cinnamon is also known to be anti-inflammatory, anti-oxidant, reduce the risk of heart disease, and provide some anti-cancer effects. For many people, it adds sweetness without the glucose elevation sugars will bring.

CRANBERRIES

Urinary tract infection anyone? Made popular due to what many have believed to be UTI prevention, cranberries are becoming an excellent addition to the diet of diabetics. Low in sugar and high in fiber, cranberries help regulate glucose levels, reduce the risk of cancer, improve blood vessel function, and strengthen the immune system. They definitely would be an excellent addition to your smoothies. FYI: Dr. Timothy Boone, PhD, vice dean of the Texas A&M Health Science Center College of Medicine in Houston states, "Cranberry juice, especially the juice concentrates you find at the grocery store, will not treat a UTI or bladder infection. It can offer more hydration and possibly wash bacteria from your body more effectively, but the active ingredient in cranberry is long gone by the time it reaches your bladder." In his study, cranberry capsules lowered the risk of UTIs by 50 percent. In the cranberry treatment group, 19 percent of patients developed a UTI, compared with 38 percent of the placebo group. In other words, don't expect cranberries added to your smoothies to work miracles for you.

GRANNY SMITH APPLES

I guess the saying is true as it relates to those green apples: "an apple a day may keep Dr. Hampton away." The research of Jaclyn London, MS, RD, CDN, nutrition director of the Good Housekeeping Research Institute, has basically found that eating Granny Smith apples can help combat chronic inflammation, which can lead to diabetes. "Apples are an excellent source of fiber and vitamin C, but are also high in water content—which can help you stay full, not to mention hydrated," says London. "I have at least one Granny Smith a day. Always."

The nutritional benefits of these types of apples include having low sugar content, high fiber, high potassium, and antioxidant properties. Remember that all apples are great options for diabetics. The best option however is the tart green apples, such as Granny Smith, because it has the lowest amount of sugar.

PEACHES

Peaches are a good source of fiber, protein, and vitamins A and C. Peaches also contain minerals such as calcium, potassium, magnesium, iron, manganese, phosphorous, zinc, and copper. They are low in calories as well.

PEARS

Pears have the highest amount of sugar of any fruit on this list, but they also have a high fiber ratio, which slows sugar digestion, making them a good option for diabetics. Pears are also a good source of vitamin D and fiber.

KIWI

If you don't mind taking the time to remove its fuzzy peel, you will be rewarded with a tasty treat that's not harmful to your diabetes. Providing a good source of potassium, fiber, and vitamin C, kiwi provides another fruit option to keep variety in your smoothie making projects.

BERRIES

Berries are a great option for diabetics because they are sweet, yet so high in fiber that they don't cause a significant rise in most diabetics' blood glucose levels. They are also loaded with phytochemicals, naturally occurring nutrients that help protect cells from damage. Another cool fact from research done on women who ate about two servings of strawberries or one serving of blueberries a week experienced less mental decline over time than peers who went without eating them. Retaining mental capacity is so important, since without it the joys of living are less. Here are the sugar contents of various berries you need to consider. Raspberries contain only 5 grams of sugar per cup. Strawberries contain only 7 grams of sugar per cup. Blackberries have only 7 grams of sugar per cup, plus more antioxidants than any other common berry. Blueberries contain 15 grams of sugar per cup. Cranberries have only 4 grams of sugar per cup. So make sure to keep berries in your freezer, or fresh if you prefer, and start reaping their many health benefits.

Diabetic-Friendly Smoothie Recipe Ideas

When considering what to put in your smoothie, it's important to be creative, with no rules other than keeping it low glycemic. Although this is not a cookbook, I wanted to make sure you had some idea of what a diabetic smoothie should look like.

Green & Orange Low Glycemic Smoothie

serves 1

ingredients

¼ – ½ avocado (adds healthy fat)
1 (4-inch) chunk of cucumber
1/2 raw whole carrot (lower glycemic index than cooked)
4 – 5 ice cubes
1 tablespoon unsweetened almond butter, sunflower seed butter, or coconut butter
1 tablespoon hemp seeds

½ – 1 teaspoon nutmeg
1 – teaspoon ground flax seed
½ – 1 teaspoon ground cinnamon
1 cup spinach or kale
⅔ cup water or unsweetened coconut or almond milk
3 – 4 drops of stevia (only if needing that sweater taste)

Keep it simple. The following example does just that:

Strawberry-Banana-Avocado

serves 2

ingredients

1/2 blender of chopped kale
1 cup of water (adjust to desired consistency)
4 – 5 ice cubes
2 medium bananas, peeled
4 cups frozen whole strawberries
1/2 avocado
1 tablespoon of chia seeds
2 tablespoons of flaxseed meal

Mixed Berry Green Smoothie

serves 2

ingredients

1/2 blender of spinach or chopped kale
1 cup of water (adjust to desired consistency)
1/2 cup parsley
4 cups mixed frozen berries
1/2 avocado
1 medium banana, peeled
2 tablespoons flax seed meal
1 tablespoon hemp seeds

These are just examples to get you started. There are no rules. The goal is to use the ingredients discussed in this chapter with a creative spirit. You will be amazed at how easy it is to drink your way to a healthier lifestyle. Keep in mind, the added fat and protein, combined with the fiber in the fruit, will reduce the impact of fruit sugars. Enjoy!

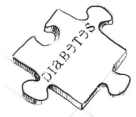

TAKEAWAYS

- Smoothies provide a great meal replacement alternative.

- Smoothies give you a unique opportunity to drink many of the foods that you know are healthy but that are difficult to get into your diet on a regular basis.

- Smoothies are convenient, high in fiber, affordable, great for weight loss, easy to digest, and high in antioxidants.

- Make sure to add healthy fats to your smoothies.

CHAPTER 9

FIX YOUR SNACKS

*"When it comes to making choices for my snacks,
my general rule of thumb is to go for the real thing over an imitation"*
~Jennifer Hudson

One of the most commonly asked questions I get from my wife, patients, and friends is what to snack on that's healthy. Most of us love snacking when watching a movie, reading a book, or just hanging out with friends. It's just a part of our culture. Most snacks are either too salty or too sweet. So how do we to resist the many temptations that would sabotage all the hard work we have been doing to stay healthy?

Remember that what you snack on is based on what you've learned over the years from your family, at work, or during play. These are not easy habits to break, but it can be done once you realize that you do have tasty alternatives. Some of these alternatives are obvious, while others will be new to you. All I ask is your commitment to not only try them out, but give them time to grow on you.

I think back when my wife and I first met. I wasn't exactly the kind of guy she was interested in, but during the year of this book's publication we celebrated our 24th year of marriage. I guess you could say I grew on her. As with any change, the key to accomplishing your goal is being prepared. This requires planning and a little common sense. So before I make some suggestions, don't forget about the value of routine.

Establish a Routine

The lack of routine is one of the main reasons we all struggle to avoid unhealthy snacking. Snacking should be a part of your meal planning and not some random act that leads to choices you later regret. Whether between breakfast and lunch, or lunch and dinner, or in the evening, snacking is safer when you plan it. My job is to give you some ideas that you may have not considered in the past. Whether it's fruit, nuts, or grapes, snacking should not be a time of regret but of guilt-free pleasure.

WATER

I have been telling my patients for years to simply listen to their bodies to determine a good time to eat. The reality, however, is that it's more complicated than that. Do most people have the capacity to distinguish between hunger and thirst? In fact, many people feel hungry right after eating a meal. You ever wonder why? The answer may be they are simply dehydrated, which leads to a feeling of thirst. Unfortunately hunger and thirst trigger the same types of signals in your brain.

This is logical to the body, since in many cases its ultimate goal is to get the needed hydration it desires. Since many of our foods give us water when they are metabolized, we get the water we need. Your body does not care that it came from solid food instead of from a liquid. The issue you face is that feeding the body's need for hydration with liquid is a better way to save some calories. Even if you ingest a food that is mostly water, like a soup or smoothie, if your brain does not feel adequate hydration has occurred, you may continue to feel hungry.

It gets more complicated, depending on how the food is ingested. Sometimes drinking versus chewing has an impact, since the brain may feel more full if it has experienced chewing. So what can you do? When you feel hungry for a snack, drink some water first.

The consequences of drinking too much water are not as severe as the consequences of overeating calorie-laden foods. Let water control your appetite. This will also ensure that you get enough fluid in your body, since so many of us fail to do this on a daily basis.

EDAMAME

This is my wife Karon's favorite snack. Edamame are immature, green soybeans harvested just before they reach the hardening period. They are an everyday part of the cuisine of Taiwan, China, Japan, Indonesia, and Hawaii. They offer many health benefits, including being high in protein and containing nine essential amino acids. They are also rich in fiber, omega-3 and omega-6 fats, vitamin K, potassium, and magnesium. They also serve as great antioxidants and have anti-inflammatory properties.

APPLES WITH PEANUT, ALMOND, SOY, OR SUNFLOWER BUTTERS

This high calorie/fat combination is a great way to curb your appetite. This combo provides monounsaturated fat, protein, and fiber. The butters provide longer-term energy, while the apple provides quicker-burning fuel, which can be just what the doctor ordered before or after exercise.

As long as you choose a natural peanut butter brand where only salt is added, you are on your way to a great snack. So make sure to read those labels so that no added sugars are present.

Also keep in mind that there are many varieties of nut butters to choose from, including almond, soy, and sunflower, so don't limit yourself. Enjoy all that Mother Nature has to offer.

FRUIT

There are many low-carb fruits you can keep in your bag or purse for a quick snack. Some of my favorites include apricots, berries, cherries, and grapes. Fruits make great stand-alone snacks, providing a quick energy boost and hydration. So the next time you are at a party and the appetizer tray has cheese and some type of fruit, don't feel guilty indulging in a little fruit. Your sugars won't complain and the fat in the cheese may slow any sugar spikes caused by the carbs in the fruit.

CARROTS

Carrots can serve as a great snack, but many of us have not given them a fair chance. It took some time for carrots to grow on me, but with time they have become an enjoyable snack. They have a high amount of soluble fiber (pectin) known to lower cholesterol, provide nutrients that lower risks for cancer, and can convert beta-carotene to vitamin A (good for eyesight). Carrots also lower insulin levels and protect the nervous system from aging, With so many benefits, it's not hard to justify at least trying to add this healthy vegetable to your list of snacks.

GUACAMOLE

With its main ingredient being avocado, incorporating this healthy fruit into your diet is incredibly beneficial. Many people assume bananas are the go-to fruit for potassium, but avocados contain more potassium than bananas. They are filled with vitamins K, C, B5, B6, and E, plus folate, potassium, and others. Seventy-seven percent of the calories in an avocado come from heart-healthy monounsaturated fatty acids, which is important since this type of fat reduces inflammation in the body. Avocados have loads of fiber, which help lower cholesterol and triglyceride levels. One very interesting fact is that avocados help in the absorption of nutrients from plant foods. This is because some nutrients are "fat soluble," meaning that they need to be combined with fat in order to be utilized (yet another way fat is helping, not hurting, us!). So the next time you need a light healthy snack, grab some guacamole or add some avocado to your salad.

RED BELL PEPPERS

This extremely healthy pepper can be used as the stick to dip in your guacamole. It is a very healthy option, and the best of the pepper varieties, since it is the highest in antioxidants like beta carotene, capsanthin, and quercetin. This pepper also contains a ton of vitamin C.

HUMMUS

How could something made of chickpeas, olive oil, lemon juice, and salt have become such a popular food in the last 15 years? The reason may be that many people are more aware of the health benefits of hummus. It helps control weight by curbing appetite, and can lower cholesterol and reduce cancer risks. It's also a great replacement for mayonnaise, and comes in many different flavors.

CHEESE

How could a book recommending a higher fat not keep reminding you about cheese? Yes, cheese in its many varieties is a great snack for low-carb eating. Packed with fat, protein, calcium, and vitamins, this extremely tasty snack is sure to be one of the most popular recommended snacks. Use it alone as a cheese stick snack or add it to help perk up the taste of other foods.

COCONUT ICE CREAM

So Delicious Coconut Milk Ice Cream with no sugar added (3 carbs) is an example of how ice cream can be eaten without the fear of carbs. No, this is not as good as the homemade ice cream my aunt once made when I was a kid, but it has a good texture and satisfies that need when the sweet tooth comes calling. Be creative with this one by adding some fruit or nuts to make it a fun healthy snack.

FLAX SNACKS

This pre-packaged snack contains only 3 carbs and can be purchased at fine stores like Whole Foods. I have been adding flax seed meal to my smoothies for years due to its many benefits. Its high fiber content can improve regularity, lower cholesterol, and reduce sugar cravings. The biggest benefit is that it's the richest source of plant-based omega-3 fatty acids, called alpha-linolenic acid (ALA), in the world!

FLAX CRACKERS

I discovered flax crackers at the grocery store, but later realized they were easy to make at home. Simply mix 2 cups ground flaxseed, 1 cup water, 1/2 tsp salt, 1/2 tsp garlic powder, and 1/2 tsp onion powder. Allow it to thicken, spread it out on parchment paper, and bake for 25 to 40 minutes in a 400-degree (F.) oven. A cheap and healthy snack can be created this way with little effort.

FULL-FAT YOGURT, PLAIN OR GREEK

Here I go again, fussing over fat. Yes, as discussed previously, fat is your friend, and when combined with carbs can slow down the sugar spikes caused by carbs that lead to insulin production, which you have learned is dangerous to your body. So when looking for a fast easy snack, avoid the low-fat options and opt for full-fat yogurt to satisfy any cravings between meals. Also remember that this dairy-derived product is packed with calcium, vitamin B-2, vitamin B-12, potassium, magnesium, and probiotics (healthy bacteria).

DARK CHOCOLATE

There are many reasons this healthy snack made from the seed of the cocoa tree should be included on your list of snacks. When you eat chocolate with a high cocoa content (70 to 85 percent) you will be ingesting fiber, iron, magnesium, copper, potassium, zinc, phosphorus, and selenium. Dark chocolate is an antioxidant, lowers cholesterol, supports brain function, and may reduce the risk of cardiovascular disease.

GREEN OR BLACK OLIVES

For the most part, the nutritional make-up of black and green olives is nearly identical. The biggest nutritional difference is that green olives contain about twice as much sodium as black olives. So, if you are concerned about blood pressure, black olives are preferred. Olives have monounsaturated fats and anti-oxidants, reducing the risk of cardiovascular disease and cancer. They are anti-inflammatory, countering the inflammatory effects of diabetes and arthritis. They are also high in iron and vitamin A (eye health). Try alone, as part of a party tray, or on top of salads.

EGGS (DEVILED OR WHOLE)

Gather your friends and family around and repeat after me: *Eggs are not the cause of heart disease!* Yes, they contain cholesterol, but research has found that eggs actually raise HDL (the good) cholesterol and even better, change LDL cholesterol from small, dense LDL (which is bad) to large LDL, which is benign.[36] In fact, there are many studies that show eggs have absolutely no association with heart disease or stroke in otherwise healthy persons.[37] Eggs have anti-oxidant properties, proteins, vitamins, minerals, good fats, various trace nutrients, and are omega-3 enriched.

Eggs are filling without having any significant effect on your blood glucose levels. I usually boil several eggs in the morning for my family and take one or two to have with my low-carb smoothie at lunch. Combined with all the great items in my smoothie, the egg adds the additional fat and protein. This not only suppresses hunger, but also prevents any carb spikes the smoothie may cause. So unless you see a rise in your cholesterol level after adding eggs back into your diet, I suggest you give eggs another try.

CELERY STICKS STUFFED WITH NUT BUTTERS (PEANUT) OR SEED BUTTERS (SUNFLOWER)

What were some of your favorite snacks when you were a kid? For me, it was Vienna sausages and crackers, or even worse hogs head cheese (also called head cheese) and crackers. When I moved into my current neighborhood and saw my neighbor's kids walking around with celery sticks as a snack, I couldn't believe my eyes. How could a kid enjoy eating celery as a snack? A striking difference in cultures! A difference that helps me understand why suggesting celery sticks for some is quite a stretch. I do, however, feel that with time our taste buds have the capacity to change, especially when coupled with the knowledge of the many benefits gained by eating healthy snacks.

Eating celery has many benefits, including reduction in inflammation, stress reduction, improved digestion, improved cholesterol, and it combats cancer. One of the ways I have enjoyed celery is by eating it with natural peanut butter. Eating good fats with your veggies is always a good idea, as I have suggested many times in this book.

SMOKED SALMON

This was one I could not resist, although it's not exactly the perfect snack. I say this because smoked salmon has a lot of sodium. With over 500 milligrams in a 3-ounce serving, it may not be the best choice for anyone with hypertension. But if blood pressure is not a big concern, a small amount of smoked salmon could be an easy way to add some healthy protein, B-complex vitamins, vitamin D, magnesium, selenium, and omega-3 fatty acids to your diet.

TOMATOES

One medium tomato only contains 3 grams sugar and many beneficial nutrients and antioxidants. It contains alpha-lipoic acid, which protects against diabetic retinopathy, as discussed in previous chapters. I find they taste best at room temperature, since refrigeration causes tomatoes to lose their flavor. I typically enjoy tomatoes alone or with hummus, yogurt dip, or with a mozzarella cheese stick. Just use your imagination and start thinking of creative ways to enjoy this healthy option.

PRAWNS

Prawns are low in calories, high in protein, and filled with vitamins B-6, B-12, and niacin. In the past, this higher cholesterol food would have been discouraged. Now with our better understanding of healthy fat content and omega-3 fatty acids, we are happy to enjoy it, knowing it actually reduces the risk of heart disease and lowers blood pressure.

TUNA

Tuna is a great way to enjoy a snack. In fact, it can also be used as a dip by adding celery, onion, mayonnaise, lemon juice, salt and pepper. Because of the many benefits of healthy fats, buying tuna in olive oil may be the best option, while also having a better taste than the version in water. So keep plenty of cans of tuna at your disposal. When you are in need of appetite curbing or a simple end-of-the-day dinner option, use tuna as one of your go-to options.

PEANUT BUTTER

You just got home, you are starving, and you were good enough not to pick up any high-carb snacks on your way home. One of the ways I reward myself is by eating a couple of spoonfuls of unsweetened peanut butter. It usually curbs my appetite while buying me the time needed to make a healthy dinner. I've already mentioned how an apple can be combined with nut and seed butters to serve as a snack as well.

CAULIFLOWER TATER TOTS

I will mention cauliflower often in this book because it can be used in so many ways. There are many recipes on line that combine cauliflower, cheese, seasoning (salt and pepper), egg, and onion to make a great tasty snack that will fool any kid trying to avoid their veggies.

Consider this same trick to create broccoli bites. How you eat your veggies will never be the same.

ROAST SEAWEED SNACK

Even though my goal is to help you change your taste buds so you are not constantly craving foods that are sweet or salty, I recognize that many of us will at times crave what we have been missing. When it comes to salt, seaweed can be a highly nutritious snack. Benefits include vitamins A, C, and B12. Seaweed also contains iodine, potassium, selenium, iron, and magnesium. This low-calorie snack could become one of those guiltless snacks that is perfect when you just get home, and is so light it won't spoil your appetite.

ATKINS BARS

I generally am not a fan of items on the shelf, but there's no denying their convenience. I therefore feel the Atkins approach to higher fat/protein with low carbs provides an easy alternative when meal prep is not possible. My favorite meal replacement bar is the chocolate peanut butter bar, which satisfies my sweet tooth and only has 3 net carbs. Combined with its 17 grams of protein and 14 grams of fat, this treat is sure to satisfy.

Keep in mind that most meal replacement bars calculate net carbs with the formula of total carbs minus fiber carbs. Atkins uses the formula of total carbs minus fiber carbs minus alcohol carbs. This is done since fiber and alcohol carbs are not fully absorbed. The key here is fully. This is particularly true for sugar alcohols. Therefore only subtracting half of the alcohol carbs is recommended, particularly for diabetes.

If you plan to use processed foods like Atkins meal replacement bars, only use them in situations where real food is not available.

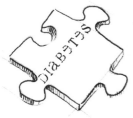

TAKEAWAYS

- Stay well hydrated to reduce your need for snacking.

- If you plan to use processed foods like Atkins meal replacement bars, only use them in situations where real food is not available.

- Make sure to keep low-carb snack options at hand for when you need them.

CHAPTER 10

FIX YOUR BREAKFAST, LUNCH, AND DINNER

"One cannot think well, love well and sleep well if one has not dined well."

~Virginia Woolf

For a diabetic, a low-carb diet is superior, since it lowers blood sugar and improves blood pressure. It has the added benefit of helping you lose weight.

This is because a low-carb diet reduces your appetite, which makes losing weight and eating this way a lot easier. It also causes the breakdown of body fat, which becomes a greater source of energy for your body.[38] So how many carbs should you target per day?

- If you don't exercise, consider 50 to 75 grams per day.

- If you want to lose weight quickly, consider 20 to 50 grams per day (ketosis range). Remember that ketosis is a metabolic process that occurs when the body does not have enough glucose for energy. Stored fats are broken down for energy, resulting in a build-up of acids called ketones within the body.

Many of my patients want more than general guidelines; they want examples of what a low-carb meal plan would look like. So here's a sample menu to get you started. Keep in mind that if you are fasting (16/8), simply skip breakfast.

A Sample Menu For a Low-Carb Diet

MONDAY
Breakfast: Vegetable egg omelet fried in coconut oil
Lunch: Green smoothie, and a handful of nuts
Dinner: Broiled salmon, grilled asparagus, and broccoli

TUESDAY
Breakfast: Full-fat yogurt and berries
Lunch: Left-over salmon and broccoli
Dinner: Baked Alaskan cod, cauliflower mashed, and lima beans

WEDNESDAY
Breakfast: Green smoothie with a handful of nuts
Lunch: Vegetarian or beef chili with/without sour cream and cheese
Dinner: Chicken tacos wrapped in lettuce

THURSDAY
Breakfast: Spinach, broccoli. and feta Crustless Quiche
Lunch: Carrot and cucumber sticks with hummus dip, with
              a handful of nuts
Dinner: Zucchini pasta with garlic, broccoli, and shrimp

FRIDAY
Breakfast: Apple with nut butter (almond, peanut, etc.)
Lunch: Lettuce wrap sandwich with turkey, tuna, or chicken
Dinner: Cauliflower shrimp fried rice with side of garlic spinach

SATURDAY
Breakfast: Smoked salmon omelet with avocado
Lunch: Salad with egg and avocado
Dinner: Cauliflower crust pizza with your favorite toppings

SUNDAY	
Breakfast:	Breakfast skillet using your favorite low-carb ingredients. *It's basically a skillet fill with your favorite low carb ingredients like bacon, sausage, eggs, avocado, and maybe some cheese and egg on top. The key is to skip the white potatoes.*
Lunch:	Tomato soup
Dinner:	Roasted chicken wings with roasted baby carrots and garlic spinach

There are so many low-carb recipes, it becomes an adventure just to discover them. I use Google and YouTube to find creative ideas. My favorite recommendation is to google *101 Healthy Low-Carb Recipes That Taste Incredible by Nutrition Authority*. You'll find many suggestions to help you along your way. I will make sure to post other suggestions on my website at drtonyhampton.com

My goal is to make sure you see the possibilities. Let's start by quenching our thirst with some recommendations about low-carb drinks.

Low-Carb Drinks

WATER

I know what you are thinking. Water seems a little boring when your taste buds are accustomed to the intense flavors in sodas, fruit juices, and sports drinks. The taste difference is real, and these high-sugar products are hard to resist. The good news is that in a relatively short amount of time, you can adjust to less sugar and appreciate the natural flavors in the drinks suggested in this section.

So how do we spruce up the most important life-sustaining liquid in our diet? Here are some suggestions:

ADD LEMON SLICES OR JUICE

I add the juice of lemon to almost every glass of water I drink. By adding lemon, you are adding folate, potassium, and vitamin C. Folate has many benefits: decreasing risks for cancer and heart disease, improving mental health, and helping prevent neural tube defects during pregnancy. Potassium helps control the electrical activity of the heart. Vitamin C is a great antioxidant and helps in the growth and repair of tissues in all parts of the body.

ADD UNSWEETENED CRANBERRY CONCENTRATE

Whether you add a minimal amount of no-sugar-added cranberry juice to your water, or even better the concentrated forms from the health food store, adding cranberry flavor to your water may provide the variety you need to avoid returning to your previous high-carb lifestyle. The benefits of cranberries are many, and include being rich in antioxidants.

ADD A COMBINATION OF FRUIT TO YOUR WATER

By being a little creative, you can become a gourmet water expert. Combine mint leaves, basil, or ginger with your choice of fruit. Although avoiding the need for a sweetener is recommended, if needed add some stevia. Consider the following combinations as a guide to help you imagine your own flavorful drinks.

Three of my favorite combinations:

- Mint leaves with watermelon

- Basil leaves with sliced lemon and strawberries

- Grated ginger with sliced pineapple

The flavor in these combinations is maximized by allowing ingredients to sit in a large jug overnight.

Try this combination to get you started:

Pineapple-Orange with Ginger

- 1/2 cup cubed pineapples

- 1/2 orange, sliced

- 1 tablespoon freshly grated ginger

If you're not quite ready to connect directly with nature, try these tips. Consider unsweetened packets made by companies like True Lemon to add a convenient, low-carb natural flavor to your water.

Also consider purchasing a fruit infuser water bottle to keep fruit-infused water on your desk at work.

UNSWEETENED TEA

If you don't regularly drink tea, I get it. It's not exactly the tastiest drink if you are drinking the usual boring options we are accustomed to. But like water, tea can be livened up with fruit and other flavors.

This is important, as tea has been found to reduce the overall risk of diabetes, and has for years been the go-to drink to help cure many medical problems. So what are some of the other benefits of tea?

A 2010 study found that green tea positively affects the eyes, protecting the retina in particular. This ensures that you'll have the capacity to see another benefit of tea, which is its ability to help all of us look younger. A 2011 study revealed that extracts in white tea inhibit wrinkle production by strengthening elastin and collagen in the skin. Black tea has been found to reduce stress and lower blood pressure. Finally, many teas have a little caffeine, which will help keep you alert as you discover new ways to enjoy healthy drinking.

A word of caution—avoid pre-made bottled tea drinks you find in the stores, as these are normally filled with added sugars. Some of these companies do provide no-sugar-added options, so read their labels.

With so many varieties of tea available, finding the right tea to satisfy your taste buds should not be difficult at all. Also consider going on line and googling flavors you are attracted to, add the word tea, and you will find someone has already made a tea that's right for you.

Or just add that flavor yourself. I even have a splash of apple cider vinegar added to some of my teas, which is a flavor I have become more comfortable with after repeated exposure.

UNSWEETENED COFFEE

If tea is simply not giving you the caffeine kick you desire, why not go to the second-highest consumed drink on the planet: coffee. Not just because it does such a great job keeping you awake, but because a 2012 study found that coffee may actually decrease your risk of developing Type 2 diabetes. It helps block a substance in the body called human islet amyloid polypeptide, which may play a role in the development of diabetes.

A large study done in 2012 found that coffee actually lowered the risk of death in individuals with conditions like heart disease and diabetes. Other benefits of coffee include a lower risk of developing dementia and a reduced risk of cancers of the skin, prostate, and the endometrium of the uterus.

With so many benefits, why is there so much confusion about coffee? Simply put, there are circumstances when coffee may not be the best option. It's all about what's right for you. So consider your personal circumstances and preferences before embarking on any particular dietary change. For example, pregnant women or people with insomnia or depression should limit their coffee consumption.

UNSWEETENED ALMOND MILK

This nut-based drink is a great way to add more nuts to your diet while also satisfying your thirst. Whether used in your smoothies or alone, almond milk is filled with vitamin E, allowing you to benefit from its antioxidant effects.

UNSWEETENED HEMP MILK

A patient came to my office asking about marijuana as a treatment option since it had just become legal in the state where I worked: Illinois. I explained to him why I didn't want to convert my clinical practice to one where I spent as much time authorizing marijuana use as I did treating diabetes. In particular, he asked about my past recommendations to put hemp powder into smoothies. He felt I was promoting the use of marijuana in that way.

I then explained to him that hemp milk does not contain THC (tetrahydrocannabinol), the chemical found in marijuana. David P. West, Ph.D., of the North American Industrial Hemp Council states that "the myth is that hemp oil is a source of THC but the reality is that the washed hemp seed contains no THC at all. The tiny amounts of THC contained in industrial hemp are in the glands of the plant itself. Sometimes, in the manufacturing process, some THC—and CBD-containing resin sticks to the seed, resulting in traces of THC in the oil that is produced. The concentration of these cannabinoids in the oil is infinitesimal. No one can get high from using hemp oil."[40]Having said that, what are the benefits of this alternative to cow's milk? Hemp provides a great source of protein, increases mental capacity, strengthens the immune system and heart, and improves skin, hair, and nail health.

I've historically purchased hemp milk from Whole Foods, health food stores, or even online with Amazon, but lately found that using the home blender was more economical. I simply combine shelled hemp seeds in a blender with water until I achieve the milk consistency I desire. I then add vanilla/chocolate flavor or stevia to taste and have a homemade version of hemp milk. Although I don't personally strain the large seed particles, using a cheese cloth to strain it may be useful for some.

CAULIFLOWER AND ZUCCHINI

My favorite recipes using cauliflower and zucchini:

Mashed Cauliflower
(alternative to white potatoes)

ingredients

1 head of cauliflower

3 tablespoons milk

1 tablespoon butter

2 tablespoons light sour cream

sea salt to taste

freshly ground black pepper to taste

directions

Rinse cauliflower.

Separate the cauliflower into florets.

Put 1 cup of water in a pot and bring to boil.

Add the cauliflower.

Cover and turn the heat to medium.

Cook the cauliflower for 10 to 15 minutes or until very tender.

Drain and discard all of the water.

Add cooked cauliflower to blender or leave in pot to
mash with masher.

Add all ingredients including the the milk, butter, sour cream, salt,
and pepper, and blend or mash to desired consistency.

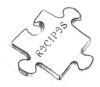

Cauliflower Rice

ingredients

1 head of cauliflower

olive oil

sea salt to taste

freshly ground black pepper to taste

directions

Cauliflower rice can be prepared in various ways: microwaved, pan-fried, or roasted in the oven. My favorite is roasting because this method helps to remove the moisture from the cauliflower, which makes it taste the closest to the rice our palates are most familiar with.

Rinse cauliflower.

Separate the cauliflower into florets, removing most of the thick core.

Add 2 to 4 chunks of cauliflower to food processor, turning these sections into rice-like chunks. A grater can be used instead, but does not work as well as the processor, leaving you with larger rice chunks.

Make sure not to over-blend, as this will result in a mashed texture.

"Rice" can then be microwaved in a heatproof bowl for 3 minutes, pan stir-fried in a little olive oil for 5 minutes, or my favorite— roasted in the oven.

Oven roasting: Drizzle olive oil on cauliflower, spread cauliflower on baking tray in a thin even layer, and roast it in a preheated oven for about 12 minutes at 200° C (400° F).

Make sure to mix it (toss it) halfway through roasting.

Season to taste with salt and pepper.

Cauliflower Pizza Crust

ingredients

1 head cauliflower, stalk removed
3/4 cup grated or shredded Parmesan
(firmer texture better for pizza crust)
1/2 teaspoon dried oregano
1/2 teaspoon dried Italian seasoning
1/2 teaspoon sea salt (only if desired)
1/4 teaspoon garlic powder
2 eggs
Pizza sauce
Toppings of your choice

directions

Preheat oven to 350° F.

Line a baking sheet with parchment paper.

Add 2 to 4 chunks of cauliflower to food processor and process until cauliflower has a rice-like texture. It's okay to over-blend a little to the texture of mashed potatoes, but not necessary. A grater can be used instead, but involves a little more work.

Steam processed cauliflower in a steamer basket and drain well.

Place on a towel to drain as much moisture as possible.
(I have found this to be the most important step to make the crust firm.)

Place cauliflower in a bowl and combine with the parmesan, oregano, Italian seasoning, salt, garlic powder, and eggs.

Transfer to the center of the baking sheet and spread into a circle, resembling a pizza crust.

Form a pizza edge by pinching the mixture around the edge.

Bake for 30 minutes.

Remove from oven and add pizza sauce.

Add desired toppings and bake an additional 10 to 15 minutes.

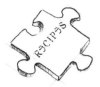

Spiralized Zucchini Noodles

ingredients

zucchini noodles (One zucchini per person usually works)

cooking spray

olive oil

sea salt to taste

freshly ground black pepper to taste

directions

Spirilize zucchini using a spirilizer.

Place a skillet over medium heat.

Add a light layer of cooking spray. Add in some olive oil.

Add in the zucchini noodles.

Toss the zucchini noodles lightly with pasta tongs and cook for 5 to 7 minutes.

(Better to have slightly crunchy noodles than soggy noodles, so don't overcook them.)

Season to taste.

Add spaghetti sauce.

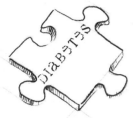

TAKEAWAYS

- Low-carb diet reduces your appetite, which makes losing weight and eating this way a lot easier.

- Create a low-carb meal plan, using the foods you currently eat that are already low-carb and replacing the ones that are high-carb with low-carb alternatives. For example, replace white mashed potatoes with mashed cauliflower.

- Drink low-carb drink alternatives like water, tea, coffee, almond milk, and hemp protein milk.

- Try some low-carb recipes.

- Once you have become an expert at making replacements for your traditional rice, mashed white potatoes, and pasta, use these as your go-to ways of preparing these sides, only eating the high-carb versions as a last resort.

CHAPTER 11

FIX YOUR BELIEFS ABOUT WHAT YOU THOUGHT WAS GOOD FOR YOU

"Life can only be understood backwards; but it must be lived forwards."
~Søren Kierkegaard

This chapter was inspired by meal replacement bars. Once upon a time I thought using meal replacement bars was a good alternative when real food options weren't available. It was a no brainer, right? Then I read the labels. It turns out that these bars are also a highly refined processed food source and inconsistent with the lessons I am trying to teach by writing this book.

What we don't want to do is to replace junk with junk. So I'll repeat what I said at the end of my snacking chapter—only use meal replacement bars as your last ditch safety net when healthier options are not available.

This chapter's goal is to give you additional knowledge about food choices you thought were good for you, but in reality aren't. As you are re-wiring how you think about food, this knowledge will help you to not be fooled by companies that are trying to capitalize on your desire to eat a healthy diet.

MEAL REPLACEMENT BARS

Food manufacturers are in the business of making money. Keeping us healthy may be on their to-do list, but rarely will that exceed the goal of making a profit. Even if they are using healthy ingredients, mass produced meal replacement bars are often combined with chemicals and highly refined ingredients. Use these only occasionally and as a last resort when you don't have access to real food. That way you won't sabotage all the hard work you've put into your low-carb lifestyle.

COMMERCIAL SMOOTHIES

After reading my chapter on smoothies you know I don't have any issues with smoothies in general. I like smoothies so much they essentially became my go-to lunch. And I didn't have any issues with commercial smoothies until I looked at the labels.

As a low-carb eater, I decided I needed to look at the carb count on my favorite brands of smoothies by a well-known manufacturer. I could not believe my eyes. The carb count was 76 grams. Although it did have 5 grams of fiber, which in theory could be subtracted, the carb count in grams was unbelievably high. Did my family really need to start their day with a drink containing 71 net carbs?

The answer is simply no. Convenient and tasty it was. Filling it wasn't. Why? Because in order to help your body feel full, you need more fiber and protein to get the job done. This smoothie had only 5 grams of fiber, 2 grams of protein, and no fat. What I thought was a healthy alternative had more sugar in it than many of the sodas we ask you to avoid. The typical soda only has about 31 grams of carbs.

I'm now an avid label reader, and these types of mistakes don't happen often. I make sure to ignore the fancy packaging and focus on the bottom line. How many grams of carbs, fat, and protein does a product have, and does it contain any artificial ingredients?

I have a simple philosophy about food: Nature has made enough of the right things to eat and there's no good reason to eat things not created by nature. Apples are okay but apple juice is not. Apple juice was often the first ingredient in commercial smoothies. Knowing that ingredient labels are organized in order of the highest percentage ingredient first down to the lowest percentage ingredient last, I realized that my smoothie was actually a juice with some puree of other ingredients added. Then I had a lightbulb moment and realized this explains why some brands don't call their drinks smoothies but instead call them juices.

I can't say they didn't attempt to speak to truth. The problem is, they were sending me mixed messages, which is why we all needed some clarification. As I have told many of my patients in the past, you don't need a list of recommended smoothie brands to choose from. You simply need to know what to focus on when reading the labels before you make a purchase.

FRUIT JUICES

Have you ever wondered why the obesity epidemic has not spared to our most precious assets—our children? One of the reasons is that they are consuming fruit juices at alarming rates. In fact, children younger than 12 account for about 18 percent of the total population, but consume 28 percent of all juice and juice drinks. There is no question that juice consumption, and the resultant increase in calories, is linked to an increased risk for children to become overweight and obese. This is also true for adults.

You've been told for years that drinking natural juice was one of the keys to a healthy diet. What you have not been told is that the average cup of juice is filled with too many calories and too many carbs. The most commonly consumed juices are orange juice and apple juice.[41] Apple juice has 28 carbs in 1 cup, while orange juice provides 26 carbs. In many ways, fruit juices could be viewed as liquid sugar, which I assume is not what you had in mind.

The real problem is that most of the fiber is taken away in the juicing process, leaving the sugary aspect of the fruit. If only we had left it in its natural state.

LOW-FAT AND FAT-FREE FOODS

Since I've written a chapter on the benefits of fat, it shouldn't surprise you that I have some issues with low-fat foods. If it were true that fat was the cause of much of the illness we face as humans, low-fat foods would be the right way to go. If eating a low-fat diet truly reduced the rates of heart disease in this country, I would put a stamp of approval on all the low-fat foods we have access to. But this simply is not the case.[42] Removing fat is not only unnecessary, it may be harmful. Many research studies are now suggesting that eating a low-fat diet may actually increase the risk of heart disease.[43] Plus when fat is removed it must be replaced with something else, which is often sugary substitutes. The problem is made worse by to the many negative effects of sugar, including increased inflammation in the body.[44] So the advice I give is to run away from products that claim to be low-fat or fat-free.

MARGARINE

Most of my colleagues follow the recommendations of the American Heart Association, which suggests that diets high in saturated fat are directly linked to elevated LDL cholesterol (bad) cholesterol. They were taught that saturated fat causes heart disease. My chapter on fixing your fear of fat, however, explains that this has been disproven, and that there is no evidence that eating saturated fat causes heart disease. It is a myth that was never proven. Old information, however, led to looking for an alternative to butter, and the winner was margarine. Many margarines were later found to contain the really bad trans fats that really are dangerous when it comes to our risk of developing heart disease. Why would manufacturers ever use trans fats? Trans fats increases the shelf life of margarine and other foods. Historically, hydrogenation (how trans fats are made) was discovered a hundred years ago when refrigeration was not available like it is today. Transportation was also less available. Hydrogenation was a miracle of sorts that allowed food to last longer without going stale or rancid. At that time, no one suspected there would be a long-term risk of artery damage. It's really a case of new knowledge/research finding an unfortunate flaw. This combined with a reluctance on the part of the food manufactures to change was likely about both money and consumer demands. Who really wants to bite into a stable cracker?

Manufacturers eventually got the message that trans fats were not the answer and now use less trans fats in many of the foods they produce. Margarine continues, however, to be packed with a lot of refined vegetable oils, which continue to make it a less attractive alternative to butter. So for my cardiology colleagues who are still looking at the data that suggest we avoid butter, I refer them to the study we have used to help us make many decisions related to heart disease. The folks who did the Framingham Heart Study showed that people who replace butter with margarine are actually more likely to die from heart disease.[45] Their conclusions suggest eating real butter and avoiding margarine is the bester way to prevent heart disease.

WHOLE WHEAT

Once grains are over-processed, they become very easy for your body to digest. This results in a quick rise in your blood sugars, which is the opposite of what we are trying to achieve. Compare the glycemic index of whole wheat bread to white bread and you will not see a big difference. They both are around 71. Keep in mind that sugar is 100. For anyone with diabetes or attempting to control their weight, 71 is absolutely too high a number.

The problem with wheat is that today's wheat is not the wheat of your great-grandparents. The new wheat is making us sick. The first problem is how it is milled, and the second is how it is cultivated and farmed. Back in the 1870s, the modern steel roller mill allowed wheat to be reduced to its purest form—white flour. The problem with this form of wheat is that it is missing vital nutrients (bran and germ), which is why it has a nearly unlimited shelf life. That's because the germ has a fat content of 10% and it's the fat that may reduce shelf-life. The current milling process replaced the previously used stone mills. Stone-ground wheat does not lose any of the wheat's components, such as the bran, germ, and endosperm. As people start to figure out these differences, more manufacturers are returning to stone-ground products. Remember, stone-ground products are much healthier than steel-cut products because the vital quality and nutrition of the grain is preserved. Although steel-cut sounds harsh, they are safe for your teeth. You can find these products at your local health food store or in the healthier section of the grocery store.

The second change that occurred with wheat occurred in the 1960s. Wheat strains were hybridized (crossed) to increase crop yields, and to make crops more resistant to disease. The result, unfortunately, was a less nutritious strain of wheat. Modern wheat is more inflammatory and raises cholesterol levels. Your take-away is simply to avoid milled wheat flour and look instead for stone-ground flour. One historical note: Traditionally folic acid is added to flour which helps to prevent birth defects. This has prevented hundreds of babies from being born or aborted every year with diseases like spina bifida. So in spite of my comments of concern from a carb perspective, flour has served our precious babies well. So the next time your indulge in some fried chicken, it's okay to feel a little less guilty if you are a women of childbearing age.

SPORTS DRINKS

Sports drinks are not necessarily bad for you. They just may not have been designed with you in mind. They were designed for world-class athletes who need to replace the electrolytes (salts) and sugars they lose during exercise. Like soft drinks, sports drinks contain more sugar than you will need while watching television, working, or even taking a walk. So until I see you at the gym or in the next U.S. Open Tennis tournament, I suggest sport drinks not be your drink of choice.

AGAVE NECTAR

When I first started my journey to find healthy food alternatives with low glycemic indexes, I thought agave nectar would be a great alternative. It does have a relatively low glycemic index. But agave syrup also contains a lot of fructose. According to Dr. Ingrid Kohlstadt, a fellow of the American College of Nutrition and an associate faculty member at Johns Hopkins School of Public Health, "Agave syrup is almost all fructose and is highly processed sugar with great marketing." She also stated, "Fructose interferes with healthy metabolism when (consumed) at higher doses." The fructose percentage of agave nectar is from 70 to 90 percent. For comparison, sugar contains 50 percent fructose, and high-fructose corn syrup contains 55 percent fructose.

BREAKFAST CEREAL

We have all been told for years that breakfast is the most important meal of the day. But you now know that due to the benefits of fasting, there is no real need to eat breakfast at all. If, however, you are a breakfast eater because you enjoy it or because you need to take your medications, it does have some benefits. If done correctly, eating a healthy breakfast can improve concentration at school or work, lower cholesterol levels, and most important, give you the energy to get through the day. But for many, breakfast has turned into an opportunity to eat more processed grains, sugars, and artificial chemicals.

Many brands of cereal are loaded with ingredients that make them unhealthy. The rule continues to be, the simpler the label, the better chance the food has had minimal processing. Here are some of the things you need to watch out for when reading cereal box labels:

Preservatives

If you see abbreviations on the ingredient list like BHA (butylated hydroxyanisole) or TBHQ (tertiary butylhydroquinone), you should be aware that many preservatives like these are linked to neurological, carcinogenic, and behavioral concerns.

Artificial Flavors

Let me ask you a familiar question. Who do you want to trust your taste buds to: Mother Nature or chemists? I do understand that maybe it's possible to go into a lab and create a flavor that would stimulate my taste buds better than something natural, but at what cost? I would prefer to live without the many side effects of artificial flavors, including headaches and fatigue.

Artificial Dyes

Go down the cereal aisle of your neighborhood grocery store and what do you see? Cereal boxes filled with pictures of brightly colored cereal which I am sure are designed to catch the attention of kids. What kid can resist the temptation of such a beautiful rainbow of colors? What parents may not be aware of, however, is that cereals made with artificial dyes have been banned in many countries outside the U.S. and have been linked to behavioral problems.

Refined Grains

I have repeated throughout this book that over-processed foods are lacking in vitamins and minerals. So what do cereal manufacturers do? They put the nutrients back in.

This is not what Mother Nature intended, and I'm not convinced that once nutrients are artificially added back to cereal that our bodies are able to use them properly. It's like eating an unhealthy snack then hoping that taking vitamins will be enough to keep you healthy. How about not eating the unhealthy snack and replacing it with real food that has the vitamins naturally within it? Doesn't that seem more logical?

Genetically Modified Ingredients

Most cereals are not organic and therefore likely contain genetically modified ingredients. This is primarily true of corn, soy, and wheat, most of which are genetically modified. The idea of eating food that has been altered from its original form is not likely to end well. Better to eat natural foods that have been minimally touched by humans. That's why so many people are using organic foods when it is within their budgets. I advise you to do the same whenever possible, recognizing you don't have to be perfect in this regard. Just move toward a better way of eating by avoiding the foods that may cause harm.

Pesticides

Most cereals are grown using an abundance of pesticides. The World Health Organization estimates that there are 3 million cases of pesticide poisonings each year and up to 220,000 deaths, primarily in developing countries. This being the case, it is important that every opportunity we have to minimize exposure to harmful substances should be taken seriously, and avoiding pesticides is no different. This is again another reason to choose organic whenever possible.

ENHANCED WATER

How did they get this one wrong? In a world filled with people looking for healthy alternatives to sports drinks, I would have expected better options. Unfortunately, instead of a healthy alternative, we ended up with enhanced beverages that are high in calories and sugars. Most enhanced water beverages have added synthetic vitamins. Researchers are still not sure if synthetic vitamins actually give the same benefits as nutrients found naturally in food.

The other problem is the sugar. Many of the beverages on the market have 20 to 40 grams of sugar, causing rising glucose and insulin levels.

POPCORN

For many of us, popcorn is an all-time favorite snack, and the smell of popcorn popping is one of the easiest for our nostrils to recognize. Since 1987, the convenience of microwave popping has become more and more popular. The price of this convenience, however, is greater than once known. Unfortunately, some popcorn manufacturers still use unhealthy trans fats (partially hydrogenated oils), which increase the risk of heart disease. And the butter used in microwave popcorns may contain artificial ingredients that could be harmful. Perhaps even worse is the chemical used to keep oil from leaking out of the bags, called perfluorooctanoic acid (PFOA). This is the same chemical used in teflon pots and pans. When heated, PFOA is linked with many negative health effects, including infertility, cancer, and other diseases in lab animals. Although no long-term studies have been conducted on humans, this substance is regarded by the Environmental Protection Agency as carcinogenic to humans.

If that's not enough, keep in mind that popcorn is not a low-carb snack and must be ingested in moderation. I suggest cooking your popcorn the old-fashioned way and avoiding the convenience of the microwave.

DRIED FRUIT

Used as an alternative to candy, dried fruit does have a place in our homes. It definitely has fiber, antioxidants, and nutrients, which are beneficial to our bodies. But as a diabetic, you need to avoid high sugar spikes and excess calories. Both may result from eating too much dried fruit. It's simply not the best option for those seeking to have a low-carb diet. So if you want to continue eating dried fruit, only eat it sparely.

SOY MILK

Only corn outranks soy as the leading crop grown in the United States. With mass production comes the use of technology and in this case more genetically modified crops. This results in a highly processed food with risks that make it less attractive as a nutrient.

I had an additional problem. As someone who is allergic to tree nuts, I was unable to enjoy a healthier milk alternative like almond milk. Soy milk was my go-to alternative to dairy. I later realized that soy milk has phytoestrogens which increase the risk for polycystic ovary disease in women, as well as cervical and breast cancers. It also increases estrogen levels in men (which I assure you I did not want).

The majority of the soy used in the U.S. is not desirable. If you're looking for a healthy soy milk, there are organic, fermented versions available that contain probiotics. These are safe and good for your gastrointestinal health, bones, brain, and healing. So use this as your go-to version of soy, or simply use almond or coconut milk instead.

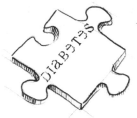

TAKEAWAYS

Always do a little research about the many foods you have taken for granted to be healthy. You may be surprised that some are not as advertised.

CHAPTER 12

FIX YOUR KNOWLEDGE ABOUT LABEL MARKETING

"The truth doesn't cost anything, but a lie could cost you everything."
~purehappylife.com

Advertising Gone Wild

What ever happened to honesty in advertising? Describing my emotions about what the food marketing industry has done to labeling, I'd use the words disappointment, amazement, and even shock. Agencies that regulate advertisers seem to have allowed too much flexibility in how definitions are used. Is a product label stating a fact or simply hiding the truth?

We should and must have a system in place where consumers are able to confidently read labels without having to read a chapter like this one to understand the nuances of label interpretation. Never take what you are reading at face value. This will minimize your chances of being harmed by what you didn't know. With this in mind, let's take a look at some advertising tricks that are used to get you to buy what they're selling.

LOW IN TRANS FATS

Advertisers now know that many of us are aware that trans fats are harmful because they raise our bad (LDL) cholesterol levels and lower our good (HDL) cholesterol levels. They have also been found to increase our risk of developing heart disease, stroke, and Type 2 diabetes.

So why would manufacturers continue you to use trans fats in their foods? Well, as I've said before, follow the money. Producing an inexpensive product with a long shelf life is exactly the combination needed to make any food product profitable. Trans fats also have a more appealing taste. So of course manufacturers want to keep you buying their products, and if it tastes great, chances are you will be back for more.

Now that the bad news about trans fats is more widely known, why do manufacturers continue using trans fats? Because they can. FDA regulations allow products with less than .5 grams of any fat per serving to be listed as 0 grams on the label. That's right, they are legally allowed to mislead you as long as they meet this criteria. The way to avoid being tricked is to watch the ingredient label. If you see a label stating 0 trans fats but an ingredient list which includes partially or fully hydrogenated oil, there are trans fats in that food.

ALL NATURAL

The website of the Federal Food and Drug Administration states the following: "From a food science perspective, it is difficult to define a food product that is 'natural' because the food has probably been processed and is no longer the product of the earth. That said, FDA has not developed a definition for use of the term natural or its derivatives. However, the agency has not objected to the use of the term if the food does not contain added color, artificial flavors, or synthetic substances."[46]

So in other words, you're on your own. When you see the word "natural," in no way should you assume that product is good for you. If you think about it another way, how many things that occur in nature can actually be harmful to you? Agave nectar is natural but contains 70-90 percent fructose, which is not exactly a healthy way for a diabetic to sweeten what they are eating. For all practical purposes, when you see the word natural, be suspicious and go to the ingredients label to evaluate what you are being sold.

NO SUGAR ADDED

Before you read one page of this book, you already knew that foods containing a lot of sugar were not good for your diabetes. You probably made an effort to avoid foods with added sugars. Advertisers know this. So they attract you to their products by stating that no sugar was added.

The problem is that many of these so-called no sugar added products contain other forms of sweeteners, which have just as many harmful effects on your body. As you know, the Federal Food and Drug Administration regulates what food manufacturers can claim on a label. According to the FDA, it is okay to use the statement "no sugar added" only when no sugar or sugar-containing ingredient is used during the processing of the food. But this does not include certain "sugars" that occur naturally in other ingredients. For example, ice cream labeled "no sugar added" may not have been sweetened with sugar, but it does contain lactose, a natural milk sugar. Your blood glucose will still spike with lactose as well.

Other examples of foods that contain natural sugars include many fruits and vegetables. So be careful to find those hidden sugars, which will still lead to elevation of your blood glucose level. Examples of high-sugar fruit are figs, grapes, mangos, pomegranates, and ripe bananas. Examples of high-sugar vegetables are beets, carrots, corn, parsnips, peas, plantain, and potatoes.

REDUCED SUGAR OR LESS SUGAR

Many of my patients believe they will do better by cutting back or eating a little less of certain foods in order to reach their goals. That logic reminds me of a person on cocaine saying they will cut back and only use a reduced amount of cocaine today. Like the drug user, many of us don't have the discipline to eat only a small amount of the addictive foods we have come to love over the years. So some caution must be used when attempting to simply reduce the foods we are so addicted to.

Look in the mirror and be honest with yourself. Do you have the will power to say no? Have you had the will power in the past? Advertisers understand that many of us approach our diets with the philosophy of "cutting back." So they make it a little easier by offering us "reduced sugar" or "less sugar" products, hoping we'll feel less guilty about indulging in these products.

You will never see the reduced sugar label on an apple or broccoli, but don't be surprised if you see it on ketchup, fruit cocktail, or ice cream. The question you should be asking yourself is, "Where was the starting point from which this so called reduction occurred?" When I reviewed the label of a leading ice cream brand with "less sugar added" on the label, half a serving of ice cream still had 17 carbs, which included 4 sugars and 8 sugar alcohols. Although not too bad (since if you're eating ice cream you already know you're cheating a bit), the message here is to recognize that you're not getting a sugar pass when you eat this product. You must be asking yourself, if they've reduced the sugars, and the ice cream still has a great sugary taste, then where did that taste come from? The answer is that the sugar is usually replaced with artificial sweeteners.

So whether it's Sucralose (Splenda) or any other artificial sweetener, you have to ask yourself if you're replacing one harmful ingredient with another. Considering all the potentially negative effects artificial sweeteners can have on your body, it seems this would not be the direction we should be moving in to live our best healthy lives.

FAT FREE

Now that you know that fat is not the enemy, I am less concerned that you'll be fooled by advertising that attempts to convince you that something is good for you just because there's no fat. While trans fats may be dangerous, saturated fats are not as harmful as we once thought. When manufacturers take out fat, they then need to replace the fat with something healthy and low in calories. This is a tricky proposition and usually doesn't end well. For the most part, the way to keep the taste in fat free products is by replacing it with sugars and artificial sweeteners, both of which are more harmful to you than the fat. So don't avoid the fat. Avoiding it will lead to replacements that make your ability to control your sugars and weight more challenging.

LIGHT

Most of us assume that light means the amount of a particular ingredient or calories will be reduced, and in many cases that's exactly what is represented when this terminology is used. The FDA agrees, and uses the term «light» or «lite» to indicate that a food has 1/3 fewer calories, 50 percent less fat, or 50 percent less sodium than a comparable product. The problem is that some manufacturers are actually referring to the flavor rather than the ingredients, as is the case with some olive oil manufacturers. Some are even referring to the color of a food like "light" brown sugar. So when you see the word "light" on a label, make sure you understand specifically what is being referred to so you can avoid being fooled by this confusing term.

WHOLE GRAIN

When it comes to whole grain, where should you give your attention? Since the ingredients are listed in order of weight from highest to lowest, it's important to see which ingredients are listed first. If a 100 percent whole grain source is the first ingredient on the list, that at least means you have the hope of eating something that's not artificial. You must keep in mind, however, that when manufacturers stopped using the steel cutting technique to process our grains and shifted to milling, we ended up with a process where we pulverize grains into a ground flour. Wheat in this state is so instantly soluble to our bodies that it's almost as bad as ingesting sugar. In fact, the carb count for 2 tablespoons of flour or cornmeal is equal to 1 tablespoon of sugar. You will never look at these two items the same way again. So whole grain is okay to use in moderation, but keep in mind that the wheat of today is not the same as the wheat of the past.

CONTAINS VITAMINS

Mama always told us to take our vitamins every morning. I hope my mom doesn't get mad at me for saying this, and I know all moms have good intentions, but the evidence suggest that when it comes to vitamins, mama was wrong. But I don't blame mama, I blame advertisers.

Advertisers know that most of us still believe that taking vitamins will make us healthy. That's why they list all those vitamins on the labels. This makes us feel better about eating what is essentially a candy bar with synthetic vitamins added. If you consider a candy bar plus a multivitamin a healthy way to start your day, then go ahead and keep eating most of the unhealthy cereal options we have. But before you do that, let's take a closer look.

About half of the population in America consumes multivitamins, and 1 in 5 of us take herbal supplements. And yet the U.S. Preventative Services Task Force doesn't recommend regular use of any multivitamin or herb. Another factor is trusting the vitamin content being advertised. Our FDA only spot-checks one percent of the 65,000 dietary supplements on the market. So why are we consuming so many vitamins? The simple answer is that there is a lot of money to be made with supplements and not so much with real food. Have you seen the cost of many of the supplements offered at the local health food store?

Although some supplements taken on an individual basis may be helpful, we need to remove the old belief that taking vitamins is necessary to be healthy. I don't want to give the impression that taking vitamins is bad altogether. This is the farthest thing from the truth. In fact, I take a high potency omega 3, vitamin D3, and probiotic daily. But I limited my consumption of vitamins after I realized most multivitamins are simply not adding anything useful to our overall health.

In fact, an article published by the Annals of Internal Medicine in December 2013 has the following summary statement: "In conclusion, β-carotene, vitamin E, and possibly high doses of vitamin A supplements are harmful. Other antioxidants, folic acid and B vitamins, and multivitamin and mineral supplements are ineffective for preventing mortality or morbidity due to major chronic diseases. Although available evidence does not rule out small benefits or harms or large benefits or harms in a small subgroup of the population, we believe that the case is closed—supplementing the diet of well-nourished adults with (most) mineral or vitamin supplements has no clear benefit and might even be harmful. These vitamins should not be used for chronic disease prevention. Enough is enough."[47] With such compelling evidence coming from one of our most respected journals, we need to rethink how we get our needed nutrients into our bodies. As stated often in this book, eating real food is the key. Our bodies and Mother Nature have a clear understanding of how to utilize the nutrients in real food. When we ask our bodies to process these manufactured vitamins, we're asking it to do what it simply was not designed to do. So stop being impressed with labels which sport the "we have nutrients" label. Just say no to what many are now calling "fortified junk food."

MULTIGRAIN AND THE CORN CONNECTION

Let's return to the theme of grains and consider wording again. We should begin this discussion with the definition of what a grain is. Dictionanary.com defines a grain as "a small, hard seed, especially the seed of a food plant such as wheat, corn, rye, oats, rice, or millet, as well as the gathered seed of food plants, especially of cereal plants."

Hold the presses! Did I just write that corn is sometimes categorized as a grain or was that a typo? Well, the answer is that a grain is defined as the harvested dry seeds or fruit of a cereal grass. It can also refer to the cereal grasses collectively. Field corn that is harvested when the seeds are dry would thus be considered a grain. Sweet corn when harvested before maturity is usually considered a vegetable. I mention this only to clarify that some of the things you consider grains may not in fact be what you are getting. Unfortunately, corn can have a tremendous impact on our blood glucose levels, so any so-called multigrain that includes corn on the list would not be a multigrain we would want.

A better way to get the grain you are looking for would be to search for words like 100 percent whole wheat. Why do we care? The reason is simple, whole grains contain the fiber we need to slow down the conversion of the grain to glucose, allowing our bodies to process them without sugar spikes. Google The Whole Grain Council's helpful chart to find terminology to help you determine what type of wording to look out for as it relates to grains. Your multigrain decisions will be made a little clearer.

CHOLESTEROL FREE

Let's start this section by you repeating after me: Fat and cholesterol are not the enemies!

Remember, FEAR again is False Evidence Appearing Real and we have been given false evidence from the past that cholesterol is harmful to our bodies. More recently, cholesterol studies using eggs as a measure of cholesterol ingestion show that dietary cholesterol has very little impact on blood cholesterol levels in about 75 percent of the population. The remaining 25 percent of the population are defined as "hyper-responders." But don't worry, since even this group's ratio to LDL to HDL does not change, which is an important way to judge if your cholesterol is actually harmful. So even this group, in many cases, doesn't actually have an increased risk of heart disease.[48]

So the idea that eating cholesterol and saturated fat raises cholesterol in our blood just does not hold water. Even if you cared about cholesterol, which advertisers believe you do, cholesterol free products don't necessary mean cholesterol free. In fact, technically there is a cut-off, just like in the trans fat category. The way it works is that cholesterol-free products must contain less than 2 mg per serving, while low-cholesterol products must contain 20 mg or less per serving. Foods that say «reduced» or «less cholesterol» need to have at least 25 percent less than comparable products. Why they allow these misleading advertising statements is perplexing to me. Are they working for us, or for the companies that make these products? My overall recommendations are as follows:

Eat as many plant-based foods as possible (cholesterol is found primarily in animal products).

Know your baseline cholesterol prior to eating a diet high in cholesterol.

If you are part of the 25 percent that are considered "hyper-responders," consider having your doctor work you up for conditions that increase your cholesterol levels, replace some saturated fats with monounsaturated fats, and eat more fiber-rich foods.

GLUTEN FREE

You see it everywhere. Gluten-free this and gluten-free that. So why the big fuss? Well, when I was in medical school, the main reason the term gluten would come up was when the professors were discussing celiac disease. In celiac disease, the immune system attacks the gluten proteins, causing an immune reaction and degeneration of the intestinal wall. When celiac disease is present, it affects the function of the intestines. An intestine that is not able to do its job of nutrient absorption results in nutrient deficiencies, ultimately resulting in other problems, including anemia, fatigue, and digestive issues.

So although it's important to make sure you don't have this condition (a simple blood test called Tissue Transglutaminase Antibodies (tTG-IgA) can help determine this), only about one percent of the population will test positive for celiac disease.

Most of us who have problems with gluten don't have celiac disease, but have a gluten sensitivity problem. Gluten-sensitive people may have problems like irritable bowel syndrome or some version of this. So for those of us who need to pay a little more attention to gluten, look for foods and products that don't have it. The good news is that the gluten-free craze has produced many tasty alternatives. If you're buying gluten-free, pay as much attention as possible to the amount of carbohydrates contained in those products.

For most us, there is no need to spend the extra money. Gluten-free products tend to have less fiber and are at times filled with other less healthy fillers that are often high in calories and fat.

MADE WITH REAL FRUIT

As parents over the years, my wife and I are guilty of caring more about our children's health than our own. So whenever we see an opportunity to give them what we perceive as healthy, we jump at the opportunity. I remember the first time I gave them a fruit rollup snack, thinking that if I could add the nutritious benefits of fruit in a tasty snack, why not? The problem is that if it sounds too good to be true, then it probably is.

I have learned that labels that say "made with real fruit" are very misleading. The FDA doesn't have any requirement about how much real fruit must be used for companies to say they have fruit in their products. Finding labels stating "made with fruit" is not only seen on fruit rollup-type snacks, but also on cereal, juice drinks, and granola bars, to name a few. So if you really want the benefits of fruit, simply go straight to the source: fruit.

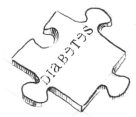

TAKEAWAYS

It's important to remember that the goal of food labeling is to sell a product, not to protect your health. Today, meals are mass-produced as efficiently as possible, which means that they are full of fillers, chemicals, and all sorts of nasty stuff. Now with a more health-conscious consumer base, food companies make claims on their packaging to get you to buy their snacks and drinks.

Don't fall for the food labeling gimmicks. Be wary of phrases like "made with whole grains," "contains vitamins," "all natural," and anything ending in "free." Use your head, check the ingredients and nutrition facts, and take note of the serving size. Your new knowledge will help you be extra safe and steer away from the products with lots of marketing gimmicks on the label.

CHAPTER **13**

FINAL THOUGHTS AND TAKEAWAYS

"Learning is not a product of schooling,
but the lifelong attempt to acquire it."
~Albert Einstein

You should be proud of yourself. You've reached the last chapter of this book filled with new ways to better control your diabetes. You've learned how to treat the actual cause of Type 2 diabetes (insulin resistance) as opposed to the symptom of diabetes (high glucose levels). This new knowledge will change many of the decisions you'll make when shopping for food or dining in a restaurant. Gone are the days when you're stuck with the choices on the menu before you. You now know the importance of asking for alternatives to the high-carb choices you normally see. Gone are the days of spending more time in the center of the grocery store filled with boring boxes of overly processed foods. You now enjoy the bright colors of the vegetables and fruits that line the outer edges of the grocery store. Gone are the days of addiction to comfort foods that make you feel great while eating them, followed by the guilt and depression you feel once the last bite of the wrong food is taken. You are a new person who understands that your life decisions are merely a reflection of your life experiences. So to make sure you are successful, this chapter will summarize some tips I feel will keep you on track as your journey to a healthier you proceeds.

The Best Person on This Planet to Put Your Faith In Is You

If we are a reflection of our life experiences, then we must be extremely aware of how we spend our time and what we put in our minds. Each and every bit of information will affect how we think, act, and behave. So the question becomes, who do you want to control how you respond to the world? Will it be you or some outside force? You already know, after reading about how food is marketed, that advertisers and manufacturers don't have any fiduciary obligations to you. So many of us have put our faith and confidence in the hands of complete strangers whose fiduciary relationship is not to you but to their shareholders. If you are not the priority, then you should not be surprised when your priorities are not the focus. Marketing departments of large companies are primarily concerned with getting your repeat business. That's what keeps their bottom line healthy. With this in mind, why would you expect anything from them other than to serve their own needs?

You must take advantage of the fact that the only person you can count on to serve your best interest 100 percent of the time is you. You will be loyal and faithful to your own needs. Therefore you must arm yourself with all the tools needed to ensure that you are living your very best life. If you have read the first twelve chapters in this book, you are already showing the desire to do exactly that. So many people are not willing to expand their brains and try another way of doing things. But that's not you. Your willingness to change and grow gives you a great advantage as you journey forward. So let's add some more pieces to the puzzle as I summarize some tips to help you through your transformation.

Become a Lifetime Learner

My decision to add "author" to my resume was primarily rooted in my love of learning. I always knew that when I learned new things, I enjoyed sharing my new knowledge with others. This came quite natural, since part of my job as a doctor is to share with patients the ways to live a healthier life. Unknown to me at the time, being a doctor gave me a vehicle to do what I was born to do, which is to teach. Writing has simply expanded my audience, and through sharing all I've learned, hopefully my ability to impact the lives of others will be even greater.

But what about you? Why should you be a lifetime learner? Well, think about all you have learned just by reading this book. In a very short time, you have learned so many alternatives to the foods that have made your glucose control almost impossible. Who would have thought that a cup of rice would contain more than 40 carbs, and that replacing it with a cup of cauliflower rice would net you 10 times fewer carbs? Such a small change, yet the benefits are tremendous. This change is only possible with new information. Imagine what you have yet to learn. Imagine how different your life will be if you stop learning. Then imagine how great your life will be as you continue to learn new and exciting ways to improve your overall health. The possibilities are endless.

The interesting aspect of this is that in order to truly trust your own judgment, you will need to know that the person you are trusting has the insight and knowledge to lead you in the right direction. This will naturally occur as you build your foundation of knowledge. Imagine being able to tell yourself it's okay to focus on eating certain foods when you can justify it with some of the research that was quoted in this book. You are now able to stand firmly on both feet, empowered with the knowledge that what you are feeding your body is based on sound, reliable evidence. That is because your trust in yourself and your judgment is not some random process that is automatic, it is earned because you have used a high standard even to evaluate your own decisions. The good news is that as you build trust and confidence in yourself, you will be able to take that trust to help you make the decisions that are in your best interest.

So stop wasting time, and make sure to spend a little time each day adding to your knowledge. I hope to be a useful resource by creating more tools to help you along the way, whether through writing, public speaking, YouTube videos, or even blogging on drtonyhampton.com. I hope to create a conversation that is not just driven by me, but includes the voices of others who can help all of us become the very best version of ourselves.

What's the next book you plan to read? Which documentary will you watch? Will you become a blogger yourself, or join the blog I have created on drtonyhampton.com? There is so much information at your disposal, it's hard to know where to begin. The only thing that matters is that you do begin, and that you become the lifelong learner you were born to be. Don't miss your opportunity to fulfill your destiny of living a long and healthy life that is primarily focused on avoiding the chronic diseases that have plagued so many people.

Start Your Day on the Right Foot and Decide if You Will Be a Healthy Breakfast Eater or a Faster

Over the years, many of us have been told that the most important meal of the day is the first one. Science is suggesting this is not necessarily the case. It may be that not eating breakfast, as described in the fasting chapter, is what's best for you. What works for you may not be what's best for the next person. I do know, however, that our lives are so busy that it's hard to have the time to focus once your day gets going. I have found if you are a breakfast person, you will have more control over what you eat when you take the time to plan in advance, allowing you to eat the right foods before you leave home. This maximizes your chances of eating the right foods and gives you the confidence to face the many temptations that exist outside your home.

So when it comes to breakfast, you need to make small changes that are convenient and simple. In fact, that's how the idea of having smoothies became so popular in my home prior to fasting. I didn't normally eat carrots, cucumber, spinach, and fruit every morning, but with smoothies it became a daily routine. As a faster, I drink a larger portion during lunch, while my family has their smoothies in the morning. Gone are the days of a quick bowl of highly processed cereal or meal replacement bars, both of which raise your blood sugars. This leads to more food cravings when the sugar spikes return to baseline, and leaves us frustrated because we feel we have no self-control. Instead, a nice smoothie was all that was needed.

Your body needs healthy fats and protein in the morning. To get extra protein, why not have Easter year round? Boil some eggs on Sunday night and then you can use them for the rest of the week as one of your go-to breakfast choices, with or without that smoothie. This is a great alternative to packaged cereal and will have a minimal impact on your blood glucose values. If boiled eggs are not your thing, simply combine your eggs with your veggies and create a healthy omelette. You can't go wrong with this type of breakfast. It will fill you up without glucose spikes and sustain you throughout the morning.

Remember your priorities. You won't be your very best for the rest of the day if you don't take care of your most valuable asset. That would be you, in case you need reminding! Keep in mind, this section was written primarily for those readers who don't plan to do intermittent fasting and want to continue having breakfast, and especially for those who need to eat to take their medications.

Never Get Your Calories or Carbs from Your Drinks

Maintaining your weight and blood sugars is hard enough when you are being asked to eat differently than you have in the past. So the last thing you want to do is to get calories from your drinks. In fact, ingesting high-sugar drinks may be the biggest source of obesity and unstable blood glucose values. Wouldn't you prefer those calories come from the solid foods you eat, which in general are more enjoyable than liquids? Of course you would. Do your brain a favor and don't confuse it with all those empty calories that make it harder for your brain to control your energy balance.

Instead of drinking sodas, sports drinks, or juices, try some alternatives that will help you instead of harming you. Whether it's water infused with fruit, water flavored with lemon, or flavored with tea, there are many alternatives that will keep you on the right track. I will always remember one of my patients who I advised to evaluate the carbs in her tea. She drank a peach-flavored tea made by a leading national brand, and discovered it had 40 carbs per serving. The bigger problem was that she was drinking this all day long and feeling good about it since she thought tea was good for her. She was partly right, since teas are a great source of anti-oxidants and do decrease your risk for many cancers. The problem arises when you combine the healthy with the unhealthy. Not only do sugared teas add calories, but those sugars also have pro-inflammatory effects that offset the benefits the tea normally provides. So be a careful consumer and realize it's always better when you brew your own teas.

If you choose teas with strong flavors like apple cinnamon, vanilla, and even chocolate mint flavors, your taste buds won't take long to adjust. I hardly ever add sugar or any other sweetener to my teas, because I only choose brands that are rich in flavor. Once you discover the world of teas, you will never go back to the sugary drinks that are harming your health. So in summary, keep it simple by doing the following:

Don't consume sodas or juices, and sports drinks but sparely.

Consume: waters infused with fruit or lemon, unsweetened but flavorful teas, and sparely drink unsweetened coffees.

Move Your Body

When I was a teen, I had the luxury of stepping outside my apartment and seeing six tennis courts staring me right in the face. As a result I spent many hours with my friends on the tennis court playing my favorite sport. During those years, I thought using sports as a way to exercise was a normal part of life, so I did not need any additional inspiration to motivate me. If only everyone had the same inspiration facing them as they walk out of their home. But inspiration is only part of the story.

There are many barriers we face that keep us from moving our bodies. What I have learned is that one of the biggest barriers to exercise is our perception that we lack the time to do it. Many of us aren't teens anymore. And our busy lives are not designed to include regular exercise.

So which is it? We don't have the time or we're not making the time? Exercise for many is simply not the priority it was in the past. But there is hope. It's all about pausing and thinking about your top priorities and recognizing that more of your goals would be possible if only you had the energy to do all you hope to do in life. So what's going to be the fuel to motivate you? You already know the benefits of eating the right foods, but what about exercise? Could exercise actually help give you the energy you need to reach your goals? The simple answer is yes. So if you are feeling fatigued and tired, you must combine healthy eating with exercise to help you reach your goals.

Research over the years has found that regular exercise can increase energy levels even among people suffering from chronic medical conditions associated with fatigue, like cancer and heart disease. Although this may seem counterintuitive, since most of us feel worse when we first start exercising, the reality is that the fatigue that follows your early exercise fades quickly. In one study published in Psychological Bulletin, the researchers analyzed 70 studies on exercise and fatigue involving more than 6,800 people. The research revealed that more than 90 percent of the studies showed that sedentary people who completed a regular exercise program reported reduced fatigue compared to groups that did not exercise.

The benefits don't stop there. Expect to experience weight loss, increased muscle, improved mood, and of course improved blood glucose control. The benefits are gained even if you start a simple walking program. Yes, there is no need to become a world-class athlete. Simply by taking a walk after dinner, you will go a long way towards achieving your health goals. So whether you start your day with a healthy breakfast or are a faster, don't forget to get your body moving so you are primed to absorb every ounce of nutrition found in the foods you are eating.

Please Start Cooking and Replacing Processed Foods with REAL Food

When I started my journey to write this book, my intention was to share tips on how to improve diabetes with diet. I knew that in order to achieve this goal, it would be necessary for my readers to cook more of the foods they eat. What I did not expect was all the other benefits of cooking that made this a very rich and rewarding experience. Here is a summary of what I have discovered.

YOU CONTROL THE CONTENT OF WHAT YOU EAT

When you cook at home, you control each and every thing you put in your body. Imagine all the things you are ingesting when you eat restaurant food, which is designed to not only satisfy your appetite but to keep you coming back for more. Restaurant food is more likely to have foods with higher content of sodium, carbs, sugars, and calories. At home you will know exactly what you are consuming, so you won't be disappointed with higher-than-expected glucose values. When you know what you're eating, you can predict the results.

CLOSER CONNECTIONS WITH FAMILY

With the wonderful convenience of restaurant food being brought to us by websites that deliver to your door, it's no surprise that many of us take advantage of all the options available to us with a simple phone call or a click of the mouse. But what are the unintended consequences of living in a world of convenience?

One is missing the bonding and connections that occur when families make meals together. If someone else prepares your meals, you miss out on making family decisions about what you all want to eat, and the bonding that occurs during these conversations. In my home, we have learned to not only make meal planning and preparing a family venture, but also try to avoid eating in isolation—that unique modern problem where everyone runs to their favorite corner of the house so they can watch their favorite television program instead of having an engaging conversation with the family. From a scientific point of view, several research studies done at the University of Michigan found that eating family meals at the dinner table was associated with fewer psychological issues and higher academic success in children. What a small price to pay to give your family a better chance at being successful. Some of the most engaging conversations I have had with my two sons have occurred in the kitchen. Whether it was while preparing the meal or eating it, cooking at home has been a vital part of what I would call a balanced and healthy family life at home. This is where most of my kids' intellectual growth has occurred.

KNOW WHAT YOU ARE EATING

What did we do before the Internet? Gone are the days when you could not figure out how to make some of the recommended healthy options discussed in this book. In fact, I always wanted to enjoy the benefits of asparagus, but lived with a family that simply didn't enjoy eating my floppy, stringy asparagus. So I decided to go to YouTube and type in how to make asparagus taste good. I found many examples of how to make this green food crispier by browning it in a pan or broiling it in the oven. This has become one of our regular veggie items, eaten as often as every week.

The Internet also makes it easy to research the benefits of eating certain foods. I've found this makes the transition to those foods easier, since your brain is more receptive to trying them with the knowledge of their many benefits. So make sure to learn as much as you can about what you are eating. Whether it's the number of vitamins, minerals, or nutrients, you will enjoy food more when you know you are making good choices. Then take that knowledge to educate someone else about what you have learned. Your knowledge will provide the inspiration others will need to make some life-changing dietary changes in their lives.

MAKE IT LAST FOREVER

In 1987, I was 19 years old and in my first year of college at Xavier in Louisiana. That same year Keith Sweat released one of his biggest singles, titled *Make It Last Forever*. Although Keith may have had other things in mind (love) when he released this popular song, the lyrics provide a way for me to encourage you to enjoy your food by ingesting it slowly.

Did you know that it may take your body up to 20 minutes to send the signals letting you know you are full? So if you tend to eat too fast, you may not have given your body enough time to feel full. But let's not end there; there are more benefits of eating slowly. A study in the January 2014 issue of *Journal of the Academy of Nutrition and Dietetics* found that you may consume fewer calories over the course of a meal when you eat slowly. Those appetite-regulating hormones that tell your brain when to stop eating need time to get their job done. Examples of these types of hormones include cholecystokinin (CCK), which is released by the intestines in response to food consumed during a meal. Another example is leptin, which is produced by fat cells and is the signal that communicates with the brain about long-range needs and satiety, based on the body's energy stores.

As we get better at understanding how our bodies work, we can then partner with our body to help achieve our overall goals of controlling our weight. The other hormone that must be mentioned is ghrelin. Produced mainly by your stomach, ghrelin is commonly known as the "hunger hormone." This is the hormone we must control, since it will make you order that desert you shouldn't be eating.

The key to allowing your hormones to work in your favor begins with the chewing process. By chewing slowly, you will give your body time to help you reduce your overall consumption. Chewing does more than break food into smaller pieces; it begins the digestion process by breaking down carbs and fat almost immediately. Chewing also sends signals to your body to prepare for the digestive process that occurs further downstream. And the more you chew, the more effective this process will be.

I'm not suggesting you take 100 chews each time you put food in your mouth (which was suggested by Horace Fletcher, a.k.a. "The Great Masticator"). I am suggesting, however, that you increase the number of chews from your current baseline, since the benefits are clear. So the next time you are sitting in front of your dinner, take a lesson from Keith Sweat and make it last forever. You may come to LOVE your new slow way of enjoying your meals, as you savor each and every bite.

REDUCE STRESS AND GET MORE SLEEP

I have so many patients who are working two jobs, many of whom have been doing this for years. Living on four hours of sleep is a recipe for disaster over the long term. I understand why people may feel the need to work this hard. Whether it's to pay off a bill or keep up with alimony payments, I get it. But reframing how those goals are achieved may lead to success. For example, when we eliminated cable from our home and converted to Internet-based entertainment like Netflix, Amazon Prime, and Hulu, we saved close to $200 per month, adding $2,400 per year to our income. For many people, that's a pay raise they would be happy to receive.

What I have tried to do personally, and advise my patients to do, is to find as many ways as possible to reduce stress by eliminating the things that cause it. In the previous example it was money, but there are many others. The benefits of stress reduction are endless. So why is lack of sleep, which leads to stress and other causes of stress, so harmful? Well, it's all about the hormone cortisol. Yes, cortisol. This is known as the stress hormone, and its elevation can lead to many problems, including elevated blood pressure, weight gain, heart disease, poor immune function, depression, and most importantly for a diabetic, elevation in glucose levels. Keep in mind this is the short list. There are many more conditions I could have listed.

Imagine having chronic elevations in this hormone because you are chronically stressed or suffering from chronic lack of sleep. The potential impact on your body is scary. So why do we release cortisol in the first place if it's so harmful in excess? The answer is that we were never designed to live without sleep or have constant stress. Cortisol, our fight-or-flight hormone, has other purposes—like helping us run from the lion or bear. The only bear or lion we seem to be running from is a boss we don't like or excessive bills that are stressing us out. Our bodies don't realize the bear is really the boss, so it makes glucose in preparation for either a "fight or flight." And if neither occurs, the extra glucose will not only increase your blood glucose levels, but will then convert any that is left unused to storage in the form of fat. So in other words, lack of sleep and stress equals worsening obesity and diabetes. So what can you do to reduce your cortisol level?

If money causes you stress, create a budget so you can see clearly what's coming in and going out. Start reducing your expenses with the goal of only keeping what's absolutely needed. Keep in mind, we thought we couldn't enjoy TV without cable, only to discover that Mohu Leaf antennas and Internet-based programs on Netflix and Amazon Prime provided enough entertainment for my two teenage boys. We even purchased the antennas refurbished on line and already had an Amazon Prime membership. This type of cost-saving thinking may allow you to either eliminate that extra job or take steps to eliminate the bills that are stressing you out. So continue to ask yourself, do I need the water service or should I make a one-time investment in a filter system? Do I really need the grass treatment service, or could I eliminate or reduce the amount I am spending on this service? When was the last time you negotiated your insurance rates? Make sure you are focused on any way to reduce your financial burdens.

EXERCISE

Now that you've gotten rid of that extra job, you have some time to reduce stress with exercise. But instead of doing something that you consider just more work, how about playing that sport you once enjoyed, like tennis, or taking a walk with your partner. Either way, you will reduce your need for cortisol when you start moving your body with increased physical activity. All you need is 20 to 30 minutes at least four days a week to have a significant impact.

MUSIC

The section in the book that encouraged eating slowly was titled Make It Last Forever, inspired by Keith Sweat's song. That song, like many others I listen to, takes me to a different place mentally. Music pays high dividends when it comes to how it can reduce your stress levels. It can remind you of happy times you like to reflect on, or it can soothe you with the nature of its rhythms. So whether it's listening to your favorite artists (my wife listens to Whitney Houston daily) or your favorite type of music (she also loves country music, being from Mississippi), you will find that music may be the key to your soul and a simple path to stress reduction. I personally like to hear the voice of Luther Vandross, whose incredible voice has been my favorite since my teen years. Whatever your taste, don't miss the benefits music can bring into your life.

MEDITATE

I am no expert on the art of meditation, but what I do know is that setting aside 5 to 15 minutes to practice mindfulness or meditation will create a sense of calm throughout your nervous system, mind, and brain. If this is done when you are feeling some stressor, the benefits are amplified even more. What a small price to pay for so many benefits.

EXPAND YOUR CIRCLE WITH THE RIGHT PEOPLE OR ACTIVITIES

Who do you like being with? What do you like doing? Why have you not talked to your favorite friend or done one of your favorite activities recently? Life can't just be about work and sleep, followed by more work and sleep. You have the power to re-engage with the activities and people who add value to your life.

- Who inspires you?

- Who encourages you?

- Who makes you laugh?

- Who motivates you?

Spend less time watching the depressing stories on the news that have you in the dumps and use that time in a more constructive way. Humans need to be connected. It's just the way we were made. If you don't have connections that are good for you, make new connections—even if with technology to connect with people via your phone, Facebook, or other means. Your day will be a whole lot richer when you share it with others. What are you waiting for? Think about who you need to reach out to and start doing this right away.

MAKE YOUR HOME YOUR SAFE ZONE

If you have issues metabolizing carbs and suffer from diabetes, obesity, or metabolic syndrome, you must make your home your safe zone. A place free of refined carbs, sugars, and other temptations that are harmful to your health and void of fiber and healthy fats. The competition outside your home is too much to overcome. They are experts on how to market the wrong foods to you. You already know how hard it is to find the right food to keep you on your path to healthy eating. So why make your home a place filled with temptation most of us could not overcome? Why market the wrong foods to yourself by putting them front and center in your home?

Did you know, based on the research by Brian Wansink, author of *Slim By Design,* that you are three times more likely to eat the first thing you see in your refrigerator. I get it. You grew up in a home where there was always a cake on the counter or where eating ice cream as the end-of-day snack was the norm. Comfort foods make you feel great and you can't imagine them not being a part of your life. I truly understand. In fact, I'm not asking you to stop eating your favorite comfort foods. Check out huffingtonpost.com to see their list of the top 25 comfort foods. Here are the top ten:

10   Chocolate pudding

9   Cheeseburgers

8   Tomato soup

7   Baked ziti (lasagna)

6   Dumplings

5   Pizza

4   Cheap, inauthentic tacos

3   Mac & cheese

2   Mashed potatoes

1   Grilled cheese[49]

How do we resist such appetizing options? Well, the first thing to do is to reduce access to them and make it a habit to eat them mainly outside your home. If I walk into my kitchen and the first thing I see is a piece of chocolate cake staring me right in the face, the probability that I will take a small bite goes up tremendously simply because it's in front of me. So keep fruit, nut butters, hummus, guacamole, and other healthy snacks—as described in the snacking chapter—within reach. Keep in mind, in order to change bad lifestyle choices into good ones, it has to become a habit first. Your first step to making healthy choices automatic is to do some spring cleaning of your kitchen and remove the temptation(s). Pretty soon, drinking water flavored with lemon and eating an apple instead of apple pie will become your new normal.

Final Comments

This book is not about dieting or eliminating any particular food group. Low-carb is not no-carb. In fact, all fruits and vegetables are carbs. Low processed food is not never eating processed foods. It's about moving towards a diet with more fruits, veggies, quality whole grains, legumes, and unprocessed meats that are natural and unrefined. Eating this way will not only help you control your blood glucose values, but will reduce your consumption of disease-causing foods and increase your consumption of disease-reducing foods. My research has taken me on a path where I now know that I don't necessarily need to be a strict vegetarian to be healthy, but can consume some meats and dairy without fear of harming my body. I do feel that authors like Dr. Dean Ornish, Dr. Caldwell Esselstyn, Dr. Joel Fuhrman, and Dr. Neal Barnard are still my heroes, because it is their research that has shown clearly that those who eat a higher percentage of foods from plant sources will likely live healthier lives. The question is, as you think about your ingestion of food, really think about it, how much will you be able to modify your diet? How can you make it more plant-based and also include the concepts I've talked about in this book? Concepts like choosing lower-carb options, healthy fats, less processed foods, and meat in its less-processed versions.

It's time to stop being the victim. You now have the knowledge that eating is an emotional experience, but you also have the power to maintain control over your own emotions. You also must stop feeling guilty every time you decide to splurge and eat those so-called forbidden foods. You are entitled to eat whatever you want periodically, and no one has the right to make moral judgments about you.

If you do treat yourself, the key is get back on track. Remember, it's not what you do in one moment but how you approach your health over all. The next time you take a trip, tell yourself it's okay to have different rules on the road. Unless you travel for a living, those trips will be few and far between and will not likely cause any harm. So don't be afraid to live a little. As long as you are growing in knowledge and your behavior reflects that new knowledge, you will find your path to being the very best version of who you are. And it will be much easier than you ever expected.

Keep in mind, as you read these last words in this book, you are not expected to have figured everything in life out by now, but instead are expected to keep learning from your experiences. You are exactly where you were supposed to be at this moment in your life. No regrets. Embrace the moment and grow from all you now know. Best wishes. Your friend and advisor.

MORE FROM DR. HAMPTON

If you want to know more about topics/articles/content/public service announcement some of which are unrelated to diabetes by Tony Hampton, MD, MBA, CPE, see below:

Content added to news service from Advocate Health Care health enews: http://www.ahchealthenews.com/page/8/?s=dr+tony+hampton&x=0&y=0

"Six myths about health that every guy should know"
from Dr. Tony Hampton of Advocate Health Care.
Dr. Hampton tells *The Patch* about the truth behind
some common men's health misnomers.
http://patch.com/illinois/chicagoheights/six-myths-health-every-guy-should-know-medical-director-advocate-health-care-dr-tony-hampton

FRONTLINE #2106
"Let's Get Married"
Air date: November 14, 2002 with correspondent Alex Kotlowitz.
Dr. Hampton and his patient were featured in this story.
http://www.pbs.org/wgbh/pages/frontline/shows/marriage/etc/script.html

"Medicare's Failure to Track Doctors Wastes Billions on Name-Brand Drugs."
Article in *ProPublica* featuring Dr, Hampton
because he keeps his patients' costs low by prescribing generics.
www.propublica.org/article/medicare-wastes-billions-on-name-brand-drugs

"Prostate cancer is the second most common cancer among men."
Dr. Tony Hampton, a family medicine physician with Advocate Medical Group in
Chicago, shares the importance of screening for this disease.
Public service announcement that ran in Chicagoland market:
https://youtu.be/fpGvLOWrwGs

"Disparities in care still undercut quality progress." (Profession). Article from
American Medical News, January 19, 2004:
https://business.highbeam.com/137033/article-1G1-166591196/
jan-19-2004-disparities-care-still-undercut-quality

CAN I ASK A FAVOR?

If you enjoyed this book and found it useful, I'd really appreciate it
if you would post a short review on Amazon.

I do read all the reviews personally so that I can continually
write what my readers are interested in.

The comments also help me grow as a writer.
Thanks for your support!

NOTES

1. https://www.ncbi.nlm.nih.gov/pmc/articles/PMC3584048/

2. http://www.livestrong.com/article/283136-how-many-teaspoons-of-sugar-are-there-in-a-can-of-coke/

3. https://en.oxforddictionaries.com/definition/belief

4. https://en.oxforddictionaries.com/definition/us/fear

5. https://www.sciencedaily.com/releases/2003/05/030522083022.htm

6. https://authoritynutrition.com/low-carb-vs-vegan-vegetarian/

7. http://www.diabetes.org/research-and-practice/patient-access-to-research/cinnamon-extract-improves.html

8. https://www.hsph.harvard.edu/nutritionsource/healthy-drinks-full-story/

9. https://www.ncbi.nlm.nih.gov/pmc/articles/PMC3946160/

10. https://www.ncbi.nlm.nih.gov/pubmed/22535969
D.L. Johannsen, N.D. Knuth, R. Huizenga, J.C. Rood, E. Ravussin, and K.D. Hall, "Metabolic slowing with massive weight loss despite preservation of fat-free mass," *Journal of Clinical Endocrinology & Metabolism* 97(7) (July 2012): 2489–96. doi: 10.1210/jc.2012-1444. Epub 2012 Apr 24. .

11. http://ajcn.nutrition.org/content/78/1/22 Abstract.
Sai Krupa Das, Susan B. Roberts, Megan A. McCrory, L.K. George Hsu, Scott A. Shikora, Joseph J. Kehayias, Gerard E. Dallal, and Edward Saltzman.

12. C. Zauner, B. Schneeweiss, A. Kranz, C. Madl, K. Ratheiser, L. Kramer, E. Roth, B. Schneider, and K. Lenz, "Resting energy expenditure in short-term starvation is increased as a result of an increase in serum norepinephrine," *American Journal of Clinical Nutrition* 71(6) (June 2000):1511–15. https://www.ncbi.nlm.nih.gov/pubmed/10837292

13. http://www.translationalres.com/article/S1931-5244(14)00200-X/fulltext

14. *Ageing Research Review* 5(3) (August 2006): 332–53. Published on line Aug. 8, 2006. doi: 10.1016/j.arr.2006.04.002. https://www.ncbi.nlm.nih.gov/pmc/articles/PMC2622429/

15. *Journal of Clinical Investigation* 81(4) (April 1988): 968–75. doi: 10.1172/JCI113450 https://www.ncbi.nlm.nih.gov/pmc/articles/PMC329619/

16. https://www.cdc.gov/nchs/fastats/leading-causes-of-death.htm

17. http://www.translationalres.com/article/S1931-5244(14)00200-X/abstract

18. C.L. Goodrick, D.K.Ingram, M.A.Reynolds, J.R.Freeman, and N.L.Cider, "Effects of Intermittent Feeding Upon Growth and Life Span in Rats," *Gerontology* 28 (1982): 233–41. Gerontology Research Center, National Institute on Aging, Baltimore City Hospitals, Baltimore, MD. DOI:10.1159/000212538. http://www.karger.com/Article/Abstract/212538

19. *Obesity* 18 (11) (November 2010): 2152–59. http://onlinelibrary.wiley.com/doi/10.1038/oby.2010.54/abstract

20. http://www.uptodate.com/contents/patient-survival-and-maintenance-dialysis

21. http://www.glycemicindex.com/about.php

22. http://www.glycemicindex.com/about.php

23. https://www.cdc.gov/nchs/fastats/leading-causes-of-death.htm

24. http://www.diabetes.org/food-and-fitness/food/what-can-i-eat/understanding-carbohy-drates/glycemic-index-and-diabetes.html

25. *Food Research International* (Impact Factor: 2.82) 56 (February 2014): 35-46. DOI: 10.1016/j.foodres.2013.12.020

26. https://www.cdc.gov/diabetes/statistics/prev/national/figbyage.htm

27. http://eatingacademy.com/category/nutrition

28. http://www.jmcphee.com/lowcarbbasics/how-and-why-it-works/

29. http://www.diabetes.org/mfa-recipes/about-our-meal-plans.html

30. http://ajcn.nutrition.org/content/75/5/951.2.full

31. G.D. Foster *et al.,* "A randomized trial of a low-carbohydrate diet for obesity," *New England Journal of Medicine* 2003.

32. F.F. Samaha *et al.,* "A low-carbohydrate as compared with a low-fat diet in severe obesity," *New England Journal of Medicine* 2003.

33. F.B. Hu, M.J. Stampfer, E.B. Rimm *et al.,* "A prospective study of egg consumption and risk of cardiovascular disease in men and women," *JAMA: The Journal of the American Medical Association* 281 (1999):1387–94.

34. M.L. Fernandez, "Dietary cholesterol provided by eggs and plasma lipoproteins in healthy populations," *Current Opinion in Clinical Nutrition and Metabolic Care* 9 (2006): 8–12.

35. L. Djousse, J.M. Gaziano, "Egg consumption and risk of heart failure in the Physicians' Health Study," *Circulation* 117 (2008): 512–16.

36. http://journals.lww.com/co-clinicalnutrition/Abstract/2006/01000/Dietary_cholesterol_provided_by_eggs_and_plasma.4.aspx

37. http://www.bmj.com/content/346/bmj.e8539

38. https://www.ncbi.nlm.nih.gov/pubmed/17228046

39. http://jamanetwork.com/journals/jama/fullarticle/205916

40. http://naihc.org/hemp_information/content/hemp.mj.html

41. https://www.ers.usda.gov/data-products/ag-and-food-statistics-charting-the-essentials/food-availability-and-consumption.aspx

42. https://authoritynutrition.com/it-aint-the-fat-people/

43. https://www.ncbi.nlm.nih.gov/pubmed/10075324

44. https://www.ncbi.nlm.nih.gov/pubmed/23594708

45. https://www.ncbi.nlm.nih.gov/pubmed/9229205

46. http://www.fda.gov/aboutfda/transparency/basics/ucm214868.htm

47. http://annals.org/aim/article/1789253/enough-enough-stop-wasting-money-vitamin-mineral-supplements *Ann Intern Med.* 2013;159(12):850-851.

48. https://www.ncbi.nlm.nih.gov/pubmed/19852882

49. http://www.huffingtonpost.com/2014/01/31/best-comfort-food_n_4698104.html

ABOUT THE AUTHOR

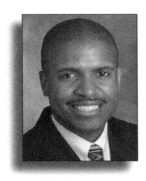 DR. TONY HAMPTON is a Family Physician who for two decades has treated patients with multiple chronic conditions. The condition that has had the greatest impact in his life has been diabetes, inspiring him to give his patients, family, and friends some useful tools to help them manage this chronic condition.

He has been a regular speaker for the American Diabetes Association, speaking at its annual Expo about "Diabetes in the African-American Community" and sharing many of the messages found in this book. His passion to empower patients with knowledge was the driving force behind his desire to write this book.

He is also the father to two young men and has been married since 1993.

Dr. Hampton currently works as a full-time physician and medical director for Advocate Medical Group in Chicago.

He regularly partners with Advocate Health Care's editorial team to write articles for *health e-news*. He also continues to engage with his readers via his website drtonyhampton.com, where he shares videos, blogs, and Twitter and Facebook posts.